Comprehensive Vascular Exposures

Comprehensive Vascular Exposures

Ronald J. Stoney, M.D., F.A.C.S.

Professor of Surgery, Emeritus
Department of Surgery
Division of Vascular Surgery
University of California, San Francisco
School of Medicine
San Francisco, California

David J. Effeney, M.B.B.S., F.R.A.C.S.

Dean, Faculty of Medicine
The University of Queensland Medical School
Herston, Queensland
Australia

Illustrations by Eileen S. Natuzzi, M.D.

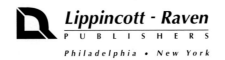

Lippincott - Raven
PUBLISHERS
Philadelphia • New York

Acquisitions Editor: Lisa McAllister
Developmental Editor: Rebecca Irwin Diehl
Manufacturing Manager: Dennis Teston
Production Manager: Cassie Moore
Production Editor: Jonathan Geffner
Cover Designer: Kevin Kall
Indexer: Kathy Pitcoff
Compositor: Lippincott–Raven Electronic Production
Produced by Phoenix Offset

Printed and bound in China

9 8 7 6 5 4 3 2 1

Library of Congress Cataloging-in-Publication Data

Stoney, Ronald J., 1934–
     Comprehensive vascular exposures / Ronald J. Stoney, David J. Effeney ; illustrations by
Eileen S. Natuzzi.
         p.   cm.
     ISBN 0-397-51342-9 (alk. paper)
     1. Blood-vessels—Surgery.   2. Blood-vessels—Anatomy.   3. Wound healing.
I. Effeney, David J.   II. Title.
     [DNLM: 1. Vascular Surgery--methods. 2. Wound Healing. WG 170 S881c 1998]
RD598.5S77 1998
617.4'13—dc21
DNLM/DLC   97-31576
For Library of Congress   CIP

In Memory of

Kathleen Lynn Stoney

Dreamer, Thinker, Doer

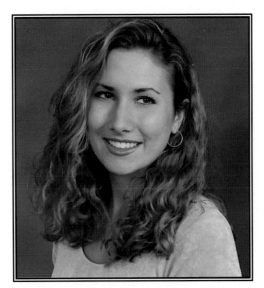

April 26, 1974 - March 15, 1997

Kathleen Lynn Stoney was an insatiable reader, a gifted writer, a Civil War history buff,
a thespian, singer, dancer, and a lover of nature and of life.
After graduating from Duke University in May of 1996 with a Bachelor of Arts in English,
she moved to St. Louis University to enter an accelerated eleven-month program to pursue her
dream of becoming a nurse. In her letter of application she wrote:

*The plane where nursing rests (that of the fundamental) is one which poses great challenges and
great rewards. Nurses immerse themselves in the most repellent and beautiful parts of life: those
dealing with the human body. It requires courage and personal strength to be able to face,
daily, the issues of death or suffering which carry our preeminent fears, and to sacrifice oneself
in the process. Yet, along with the possibility for despair comes one for deepest joy,
and nursing bestows the honors that accompany the mysteries of life.
There is birth in nursing and renewal and hope.*

On May 16, 1997, Kathleen Lynn Stoney was recognized as a Daughter of St. Louis University
School of Nursing for personifying the ideals expressed in their Mission Statement.

Contents

Preface

Comprehensive Vascular Exposure is a single volume designed to present exposure of vascular structures as a dynamic process of wound engineering that results in an environment that will optimize healing of the vascular reconstruction. This concept is the result of experience derived over four decades of providing vascular surgical treatment of patients at the University of California, San Francisco. The chapters begin with the application of the principles of exposure and then, in sequence, review the exposure of eight specific anatomic body regions, concluding with a chapter on tunnels, a specialized wound often considered important. The volume features a concise text liberally illustrated with full-sized, detailed, full-color drawings and operative photographs to demonstrate the wound engineering required to achieve optimal healing of the vascular repair.

Ronald J. Stoney, M.D.
David J. Effeney, M.B.B.S.

Acknowledgment

To have the opportunity to write, illustrate, and have a book published is a rare privilege. We are grateful to many who have eased the task of completing this work.

Eileen Natuzzi, M.D., has combined her knowledge and skill as a physician, surgical resident, and vascular surgical trainee with her remarkable talent and experience in medical illustration to bring the text to life with precision, clarity, and meaning through her comprehensive illustrative work.

Ronald J. Stoney, M.D.
David J. Effeney, M.B.B.S.

1
A Thesis

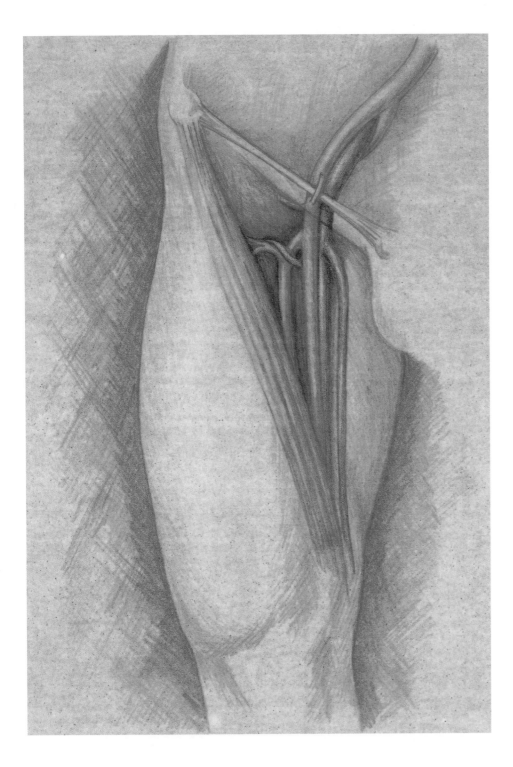

Webster defines the term exposure in both an active and a passive voice: "To set forth, to be open to view." The word is derived from the Latin *exponere,* meaning to set out, and of course it has other meanings in modern English usage.

When applied to the science and art of surgery, the term exposure has classically meant the extent of dissection required to perform a surgical procedure or the confirmation or denial of an operative diagnosis. The procedure was the dominant feature of early training in surgery; all of us were beguiled by the extent of possible resection of organs and eventually replacement of arteries. The practical demonstration of bypass by Kunlin in the 1940s added further to the excitement felt by "vascular surgeons." The extended scope of many procedures was made possible by increasing knowledge and technological advances.

This focus on the procedure was reflected in our documentation of any operation in which we reduced our thinking about the process to a series of four major categories:

- Incision
- Pathology/findings
- Procedure
- Closure

We wrote our operative notes accordingly.

The term "exposure" was used only rarely but was well understood by the master surgeons. Ross Dunn, in his blunt colonial way, best summarized it with his classic quote, "If you can bloody well see it, you can bloody well do it." Jack Wylie would beseech us "to get a bit more artery to work with" when we thought we had enough.

The technological revolution has continued. The adaptation of the early laparoscope from a single-dimension instrument to a widely used sophisticated system of specialized and integrated instruments has caused us all to review our concepts of exposure. For a successful and safe cholecystectomy, it was once *de rigueur* to make a relatively large incision in order to adequately visualize the gallbladder and biliary tree, which were held "in view" by two assistants displacing the gut and liver and rotating the free edge of the liver so that the edge of the lesser omentum was brought onto the stretch. The nature of this procedure required an 8- or 9-inch abdominal wall wound. The most important operative step was the placement of the first assistant's left hand to gain and hold "exposure."

Now exposure is generated by CO_2 insufflation of the abdominal cavity with four to five band-aid-sized wounds providing access. Retention of the viscera is accomplished by the increased intraabdominal pressure and the positioning of the patient. The displacement of the liver is achieved more easily with the abdomen closed and distended with gas than with an open peritoneal cavity. Visualization of the critical areas is achieved with the use of a cold light source and optic fibers to deliver the light accurately; a high-resolution video camera and color monitor complete the setup. Exposure for cholecystectomy has been totally reengineered.

Although the four-point operative note system had the perceived virtue of clarity and was easy to follow, it obscured the fact that the accurate delineation of the pathology, the accurate performance of the procedure, and the closure of the wound were all dependent on the original exposure obtained.

The story in vascular surgery is much the same as these examples from general surgery. The technological revolution has resulted in more versatile and generally superior grafts, more specifically designed instruments, and much improved suture technology, particularly needle technology. The rapid advances in technology have been coupled with a better understanding of arterial wall biology and of the response of the arterial wall to atherosclerosis. More importantly, we are at last beginning to understand how the arterial wall responds when injured during vascular repairs after endarterectomy and following the attachment of prosthetic grafts. All of these advances have benefited our patients when vascular surgery is well performed for appropriate indications.

Those of us who have had the privilege of taking care of numbers of patients and watching them return for follow-up visits have noted that the patients who did well in general terms were those who had no healing complications. Again, in general terms, their vascular procedures were free from technical problems, and the initial "responses to injury" of the vascular wound were short-lived in duration and self-limiting in progression. When these patients had endarterectomies, the vessel wall had minimal myointimal hyperplasia in the operated segment. Those with grafts had well-incorporated grafts separated from other vital structures, particularly the hollow organs.

These observations have prompted a search for the reasons why it should be so. The thesis that appeals to us is that the original exposure and conduct of the index vascular repair were of high caliber, resulting in a lack of healing complications, the progression of which could have led to ultimate failure of a reconstruction.

The opportunities to reoperate on a number of patients have been informative and persuasive in leading us more and more to accept this thesis. Initially, the anatomic areas involved in failures of primary reconstructions were avoided. These "no go" areas were bypassed and excluded. Direct reoperation on previously endarterectomized arteries was thought to be highly undesirable and technically difficult. A failed prosthetic graft might well be replaced with some form of extraanatomic bypass. Only when we reoperated directly on the failed reconstruction through the original wound and saw our own and other surgeons' handiwork did we fully comprehend the extent to which "the exposure" or "lack of exposure" or "perversion of exposure" led to healing complications and reconstruction failure. The concept of "wound engineering" in vascular surgery was clearly relevant to an increased knowledge of how to prevent the early healing complications that predispose the patient to reconstruction failure.

Vascular exposure thus has taken on a broader meaning than the mere display of the vessels to be operated upon. It is certainly not a passive process. For the purpose of this volume, we propose to use the term *exposure* to mean "the wound engineering required to create an environment for optimal healing of a vascular reconstruction."

We do not intend to describe or illustrate any particular vascular operation *per se*—we have previously attempted to do that. Rather, we propose to develop the principles we see encompassed by the definition of exposure by application to each anatomic region that is a common site of vascular exposure, then to systematically review the relevant anatomy and describe the exposure of major areas of interest to the vascular surgeon. The tools we propose to use are the written word, anatomic and operative photography, and the skilled illustrations of Eileen Natuzzi, M.D.

The definition of exposure we have adopted as a thesis should of course be subject to vigorous questioning and criticism—a process we have followed for ourselves during the genesis of this work. We acknowledge the contributions of many others to our thinking on these matters but believe we should put forward the views we currently hold as our own and thus do not include formal references to the work of other scientists and surgeons.

A major vascular operation consists of a well-thought-out, coherent series of steps that follow logically one upon the other. From the incision of the skin to the insertion of the final suture, an operation is a process. Any process can be reengineered to make it better, more efficient, and able to produce better outcomes, and output can be improved by the deleting unnecessary steps.

The process of wound engineering is an active one, initiated and carried through by an individual surgeon. Thus, the processes must allow for modification to suit surgeon preference and capability. An incision along the anterior border of the sternocleidomastoid in the neck to expose the carotid artery bifurcation is as valid as a more transverse incision following a skin crease immediately over the bifurcation. The debate about which incision is better may have been prolonged and at times passionate, with neither party to the debate being likely to be won over on the respective merits of his or her counterpart's argument. However, in the big picture of engineering the wound to allow the endarterectomized vessel optimal healing, the choice of the direction of the skin incision is almost irrelevant. Both incisions heal well with cosmetically acceptable results. More important is the capability of the surgeon to place the incision to gain access to the appropriate tissue planes so that muscle bellies are not violated during the construction and development of the "route to the vessels."

The wound must be fashioned to allow the skin edges to be retracted and the deeper structures to be retained safely out of the operative field of view. Sufficient lengths of the vessels must be exposed for safe clamping above and below the intended area of vascular wounding. Sufficient space must be generated around the vessels to allow the safe accomplishment of the technical procedures of the operation.

In addition, there is a requirement for the surgeon to plan to be able to perform an alternative repair if the primary operation proposed proves not to be feasible or in the rare event of a major technical misadventure.

The wound created for any operation will thus depend on the patient's habitus and the position into which he or she can be moved; the route chosen to gain access to the vessels; the pathology to be dealt with; the site, type, and distribution of the vascular disease; and the individual preference of the operating surgeon.

The wound must be created in a way that ensures the viability of the vessel, with both the nutritional status and the nervous innervation of the vessel maintained. The periarterial tissue must be viable, a result brought about by the correct choice of tissue planes that do not cut across vascular supply, venous or lymphatic drainage, and innervation. Any obviously devitalized or suspect tissue should be excised at any level along the route of access to the vessels within an operative or traumatic wound but particularly in the periarterial region. The wound should be engineered so that any prosthetic material is accommodated comfortably, surrounded by and in direct contact with viable well-perfused tissues.

The restoration of the properly engineered wound should result in close approximation of tissue layers, held without tension, to obliterate potential dead space. We must aim to prevent accumulation of blood, lymph, and chyle at all levels in the wound. This is the mechanical engineering of infection prevention, one of the key outcomes of this whole process.

When it is not possible to completely obliterate the dead space mechanically by apposition, or if there is any risk of fluid accumulation at any level in the wound, then we believe closed-system suction drainage should be used to ensure that there is no fluid accumulation that separates the artery from surrounding viable tissue or separates tissue layers. This represents some change from what might have been interpreted from our previous writings. However, the shift is a measure of our belief in creating the optimal environment for vascular wound. The risks of closed-system suction drains used for the short term are much less than the risks of dead space and fluid accumulation as far as major complications of healing are concerned, especially those related to wound hypoxia and infection.

In addition, there are some wounds—the harvest site of the long saphenous vein and the reoperative wound—that are very prone to fluid accumulation and the production of dead space with subsequent morbidity. These wounds should be drained routinely as well.

Tunnels are used frequently in vascular surgery. They are specialized wounds designed to connect two sites of open vascular display. This type of wound has been very much underestimated and is not often considered as an aspect of exposure. Yet, tunnels are quite frequently the source of morbidity, altered healing, and long-term problems for the patient.

Tunnels are created in various body spaces or potential spaces—subcutaneous, retroperitoneal, submuscular, or interfascial body compartments. They may be anatomic in the sense that they follow a path of a named neurovascular bundle or extraanatomic when the tunnel is remote from the artery the conduit it contains will replace. These tunnels are inarguably a wound and an important component of the concept of exposure even though there may be no exposed artery or arterial wounds in their length.

Tunnels may traverse a variety of structures, often more than one body region, and they not infrequently cross sites of active motion. Because of this, correct tunneling requires careful attention to the procedures of planning, precision, and restoration described previously. Atraumatic instrumentation along well-defined routes should be the norm. The routes chosen should avoid areas where leakage of lymph or predictable bleeding from arterial or venous damage will be a problem. The concerns about tunnels are generally more significant in reoperative surgery, where the tunnel may be the most significant part of the procedure requiring the engineering of a new wound in viable tissue even though the scar of a previous incision and access route may have been reopened.

This text then is an attempt to develop further our own belief that comprehensive vascular exposure can be thought of as creating an optimal environment for the healing of a vascular reconstruction. The exposure includes the display of the sites of interest to the surgeon and prepares for the restoration of the wound after the operative intervention.

There are, however, in our minds, a defined hierarchy of areas for healing:

1. The vascular wound.
2. The perivascular structures.
3. The routes of access to the vessels.
4. The skin.

Further, there are developed concepts that would allow the wound engineering to proceed in any wound. These include:

1. The planning of the exposure.
2. The protection of the patient, the vessels, and other structures at risk in the operative field.
3. The creation of the incision and routes of access to the vessel.
4. The precise performance of the vascular reconstruction.
5. The restoration of exposure to as near normal as is practical.

So far in this discussion we have focused broadly on concepts and principles we have adopted based on the observation of our own patients followed over many years. We have become persuaded by these observations that the wound environment that results after a surgical procedure is the key determinant of rapid complication-free healing. We have been surprised when we looked for technical errors in patients with early but not acute reconstruction failures that these errors were not always obvious. Improvement of technical expertise and the increasing use of intraoperative methods to detect correctable technical errors have been major advances and have led to significant diminution worldwide in the incidence of acute reconstructive failure.

We are persuaded that many of the complications after an arterial repair are caused by the exposure itself. Some complications, such as bleeding or thrombosis, develop early and are obvious. However, the later complications of myointimal hyperplasia and the progression of atherosclerosis in the areas of vascular reconstruction are the more subtle but pervasive outcomes of the healing perversions in suboptimal wound environments.

The basic biology of these observations is under investigation on a worldwide basis as surgeons, scientists, and vascular biologists have moved from the mechanical and technical problems now largely understood, if not solved, to try and understand what Alan Callow so graphically described as the "microcosm of the arterial wall."

For us, the ultimate challenge is to provide a healing environment that controls and regulates the behavior of the arterial smooth muscle cell in the injured arterial wall. The control of the phenotypic change necessary for initial repair after vascular wounding and the rapid reversion from the secretory and proliferative mode of the smooth muscle cells are products of the local environment. We believe that provision of the optimal healing environment is a product of the careful design and conduct of a comprehensive vascular exposure.

2

Practical Application of the Principles

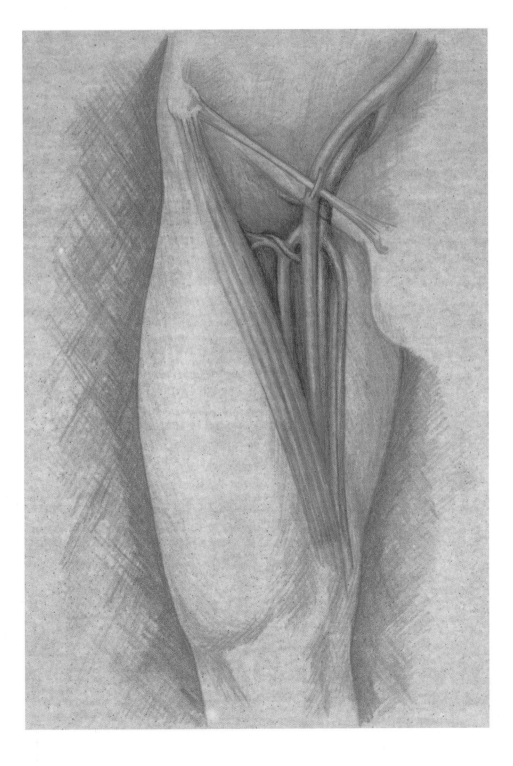

In this chapter we use a region of the body commonly entered by vascular surgeons—the groin—to explore the principles we have developed about exposure.

SURGICAL ANATOMY OF THE COMMON FEMORAL ARTERY AND ITS MAJOR BRANCHES

The common femoral artery is the continuation of the external iliac artery and shares with the proximal internal carotid artery the distinction of being the only two major arteries that are larger than their vessels of origin. Anatomically the common femoral artery begins behind the inguinal ligament and enters the femoral triangle at about the midpoint of its base. The vessel divides within the triangle to form the superficial femoral and profunda femoris arteries. The superficial femoral artery crosses the triangle and exits through the apex to enter the subsartorial canal. In life, the femoral triangle corresponds to the depression below the groin crease (see chapter-opening art on page 7). The triangle is formed by the inguinal ligament above, the medial border of sartorius muscle, and the medial border of adductor longus. The floor of the triangle, which has a trough or gutter shape, is formed from above down and from lateral to medial by four muscles: iliacus, psoas major, pectineus, and adductor longus. The common femoral artery is related posteriorly to the psoas and pectineus muscles.

The contents of the femoral triangle are the femoral vessels, which lie in the deepest part of the trough, the branches of the femoral nerve, lymph nodes and fat (Fig. 2-2). The external iliac artery begins at the bifurcation of the common iliac artery at about the brim of the true pelvis; it runs downward and laterally along the medial bor-

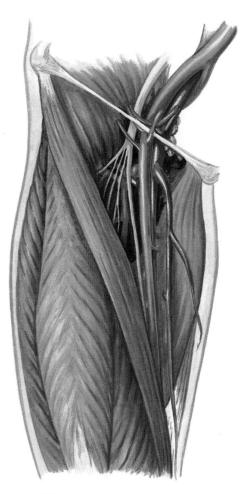

Figure 2-2. The anatomy of the groin.

der of the psoas major muscle, separated from the muscle by the iliac fascia. In front of the vessel and medially, there is a direct relationship of the artery to the parietal peritoneum, extraperitoneal fat, and the other extraperitoneal tissues. There are also numerous lymph nodes and abundant lymph channels, which may cause troublesome lymph leaks after mobilization of structures in this area and require serious consideration by the surgeon when constructing a retroperitoneal tunnel. The vessel has no major branches until its termination, where the inferior epigastric and the deep circumflex iliac arteries are given off. Above these two branches the external iliac artery is crossed by the lateral circumflex iliac vein—"the vein of sorrow"—shortly before that vein enters into the external iliac vein.

The common femoral artery is enclosed for the first few centimeters of its length within the femoral sheath, a fascial condensation and inferior extension of the iliac fascia posteriorly and the transversalis fascia anteriorly. It is usually thought of as having (from lateral to medial) three compartments: an arterial compartment containing the femoral artery and the femoral branch of the genitofemoral nerve; a venous compartment containing the femoral vein; and the potential space called the femoral canal, which contains fat and the lymph node of Cloquet. The sheath is well developed and is readily separated over the proximal common femoral artery but blends with the periarterial tissue toward and beyond the bifurcation of the common femoral artery (Fig. 2-3).

The common femoral artery branches into two major vessels. The superficial femoral artery is usually the larger of the two branches and is the arterial conduit that carries blood to the leg. The profunda femoris artery is the artery of supply to the tissues of the thigh.

As stated earlier, the superficial femoral artery passes through the femoral triangle and exits into the subsartorial canal by passing through the musculofascial apex of the femoral triangle. This canal extends from the apex of the femoral triangle to the adductor hiatus in adductor magnus muscle, through which it gains access to the popliteal space and becomes the popliteal artery. The subsartorial space appears somewhat triangular when the thigh is seen in cross section and is bordered by the sartorius muscle medially, the vastus medialis anterolaterally, and the adductor muscles, initially adductor longus and subsequently adductor magnus, posteriorly.

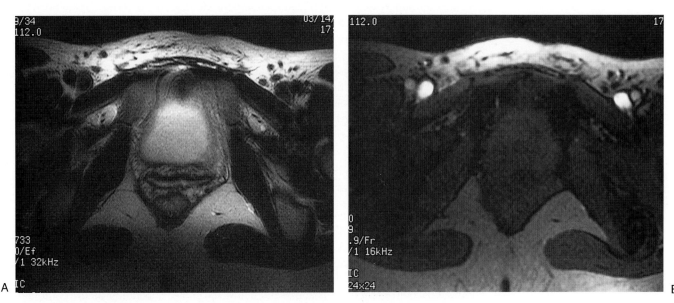

Figure 2-3. Magnetic resonance image of cross section of groin. **A:** Fast spin-echo T$_2$ showing flow voids in femoral artery and vein. **B:** Axial gradient echo showing venous blood as brighter than adjacent artery.

The profunda femoris artery arises from the posterolateral aspect of the common femoral. The medial and lateral circumflex femoral vessels are given off as branches soon after its origin, although in about 20% of patients these vessels arise from the common femoral artery at the level of the bifurcation. These arteries are important collaterals that can function in either direction, being the reentry vessels from the cruciate anastomosis around the hip when the external iliac artery is narrowed or occluded and the supplying vessels to the cruciate anastomosis when the internal iliac artery is severely diseased. The lateral circumflex femoral branch has ascending and descending branches, the latter of which runs along the vastus lateralis to the knee.

The profunda femoris artery usually has three perforating arteries that supply the musculature of the thigh, and the profunda ends by piercing adductor magnus in what is sometimes called the fourth perforating branch. The first perforating artery has an ascending and a descending branch, whereas the other perforating vessels are connected by a rich anastomotic network. Besides the perforating branches, there are several large muscular branches that anastomose in the medial compartment in the thigh to form a series of anastomotic vessels that are parallel to the perforators. At the lower end of the artery, the medial collateral branches anastomose with popliteal muscular branches, particularly the medial superior geniculate artery. The lateral collateral pathway anastomoses with the lateral superior geniculate muscular branches. Through the geniculate system around the knee joint, these profunda branches carry blood to the tibial recurrent and upper muscular branches of the main crural arteries when the popliteal artery is occluded. Thus, the profunda femoris collateral system has the capacity to bring blood from the cruciate anastomosis around the hip joint to the tibial vessels.

Shortly after the bifurcation of the common femoral artery, the profunda femoris artery passes behind the lateral border of adductor longus and is covered by that muscle. Posteriorly from above to below, the artery lies on pectineus muscle, adductor brevis, and adductor magnus.

Immediately below the bifurcation of the common femoral artery, the profunda femoris is crossed by the lateral circumflex femoral vein just before that major tributary enters the common femoral vein.

Within the femoral triangle, the common femoral artery and its bifurcation are surrounded by lymph channels, and above the femoral sheath and deep to the fascia lata, the deep inguinal nodes are found medial to the common femoral vein. Above the fascia lata, the superficial nodes lie lateral to where the main trunk of the saphenous vein enters the fossa ovalis and are in an immediate anterior relationship to the artery. They are at risk of injury during the incision and development of the route of access to the artery. These nodes are contained in the superficial fascia, which, in the region of the groin, has a well-developed membranous layer. The superficial fascia of the groin is also known as Camper's fascia.

The anatomy of the groin region determines the method of exposure of the common femoral vessels, the route of access to the arteries, and the closure required to conform to principles we asserted previously. The anatomy also dictates how and where the tunnels entering and leaving this region should be begun or ended.

EXPOSURE IN THE FEMORAL TRIANGLE

The patient should be positioned supine. The legs should be well supported, and the heels positioned so that they are about 30 cm apart. The feet are allowed to rotate externally.

A vertical or slightly curved linear skin incision is made directly over the common femoral artery (Fig. 2-4). This incision crosses the groin crease for all groin exposures but will have different lengths above and below the crease depending on the pathology to be overcome and the purpose of the proposed procedure. For most aortofemoral grafting procedures to a relatively undiseased femoral system, the skin crease repre-

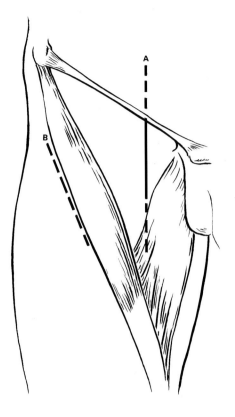

Figure 2-4. Illustration of the proximal thigh depicting a vertical incision A (*dotted and solid lines*) and oblique incision B (*dotted lines*). A is used in femoral bifurcation exposures. B is used in distala exposure of profunda femoris artery.

sents the middle of the wound. For femoropopliteal and profunda reconstructions, the length below the groin crease will be considerably greater than that above.

When a pulse is present at the common femoral artery, the incision is placed accordingly. When a pulse is absent, the incision should pass through a point on the inguinal ligament that is midway between the anterior superior iliac spine and the pubic symphysis—the so-called midinguinal point. This incision is made with a sharp scalpel,

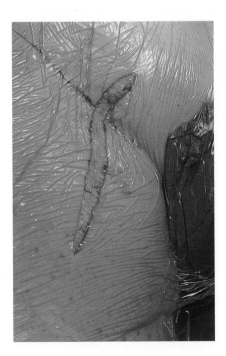

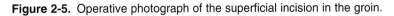

Figure 2-5. Operative photograph of the superficial incision in the groin.

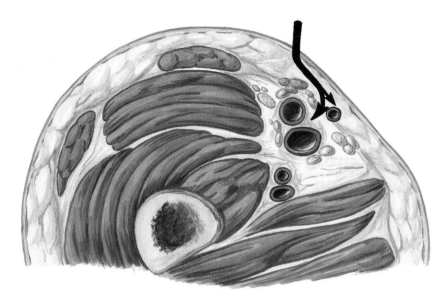

Figure 2-6. Route of access through the groin incision to the femoral vessels.

and the skin is divided cleanly; the blade should be held at right angles to the skin throughout the length of the cut. The skin is held at the appropriate tension by the surgeon and first assistant during the performance of the initial incision (Fig. 2-5).

The wound may be developed further by sharp dissection using a scalpel to divide through the superficial fascia, avoiding the lymph nodes (Fig. 2-6). Any lymphatic trunks should be coagulated to prevent lymph leaks. The only superficial structures

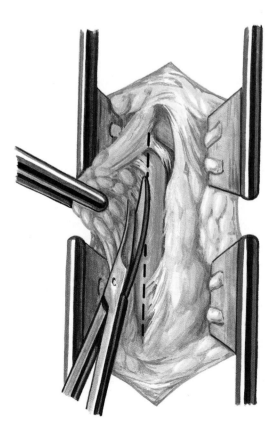

Figure 2-7. Deeper exposure with retraction and separation of lymphatics and exposure of fascia.

apart from the lymph nodes and vessels are one or two superficial veins that cross in front of the common femoral artery, coursing from lateral to medial to join the long saphenous vein in the fossa ovalis. These veins should be ligated. This dissection proceeds with a clean incision to expose the femoral sheath, the inguinal ligament, and the lower fibers of the external oblique muscle (Fig. 2-7).

An alternative methodology uses diathermy with blended cutting and coagulating currents. The skin edges are elevated and separated by hand-held rake-type retractors, and the diathermy needle is used to divide the tissue. The surgeon and assistant each hold a retractor and apply sufficient traction and countertraction to the skin edges to present the tissue for division. This method facilitates avoidance of the major lymph nodes and produces a dry wound. The superficial venous tributaries are dealt with by ligation.

Once the anterior lamella of the femoral sheath over the common femoral artery is on display, standard scissors and forceps dissection is used after the appropriate skin edge retraction and soft tissue retention have been established.

Retractors

We favor self-retaining retractor systems, as they provide better and more stable visualization than hand-held retractors. We are not persuaded that prolonged periods of retractor holding contribute to surgical education, nor should it be considered a potential rite of passage to advancement in surgical training (Fig. 2-8).

The main reason, however, for using self-retaining systems is simply put: they are better. They provide better visualization and produce a stable operative field. There is no fatigue. When the systems are chosen and used appropriately, there is less damage to the skin and soft tissues.

Various types of retractor systems are available. We use the wishbone table-mounted system, which is eminently suitable and enables all the required maneuvers to be accomplished in any groin operation. When wishbone systems are not available, the older, spreading, ratchet-type retractors are still suitable. We tend to use two retractors for each groin wound. The retractor lying along the thigh has straight handles, and the retractor that is inserted in the upper part of the wound has a handle with hinges in the middle of its length to enable conformity to the abdominal contours. These retractors lie well in the wound, and the use of two retractors spreads the tension of the skin and subcutaneous tissue more evenly while producing significantly better visualization as the wound adopts a more rectangular profile rather than the diamond shape achieved by a single self-retaining device. A hand-held retractor of the Langenbeck type is useful in elevating the inguinal ligament when the external circumflex iliac vein is ligated and divided.

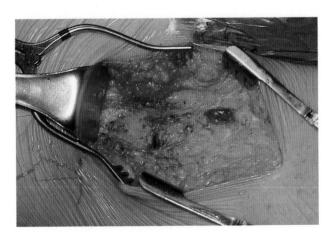

Figure 2-8. Operative photograph showing superficial exposure and retraction of groin.

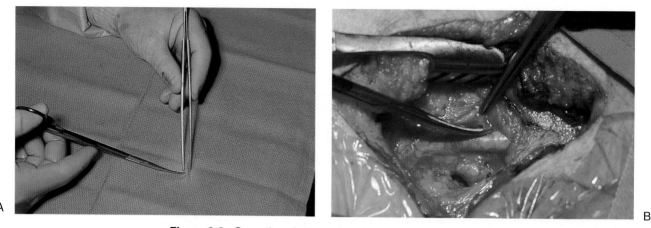

Figure 2-9. Operative photographs of scissors and forceps dissection required to conduct precise exposure of the vessels.

Scissors and Forceps Dissection

Satisfactory retraction and soft-tissue retention facilitate the final exposure of the common femoral artery. We use blunt, round-pointed Metzenbaum scissors. These scissors have nicely rounded ends that transmit through the blades and handles a strong sensation of the quality of the tissue being spread and cut. We avoid sharp-pointed scissors because they are dangerous and do not allow the technique of spreading and dissection to be accomplished with safety (Fig. 2-9).

We use two pairs of broad-tipped forceps, held by the assistant and surgeon, to provide the traction and countertraction while the scissors blade spreads and divides between the instruments. We prefer to use the smooth wide forceps and favor standard student thumb forceps, which are very satisfactory in the dissection and for holding the arterial walls. Once the surgeon gets used to these rather old-fashioned instruments, they are easy and comfortable to use. Fine, strongly grasping forceps must be avoided, particularly when handling the vessel wall; they inflict small focal areas of crush injury to fat and any other tissues they grasp.

During forceps and scissors dissection, the surgeon holds the forceps in his or her left hand and the scissors in the other. The assistant should hold the forceps in the left hand and a suction tip in the right hand. The surgeon picks up the tissue just to his or her side of the proposed line of incision, and the assistant picks the tissue up directly opposite with a distance of about 5 to 6 mm between the two forceps. Both elevate and lift the tissue to provide the tension, traction and countertraction, while the surgeon applies the slightly spread points of the scissors to the tissue, gauges the tissue's quality, and then incises that area. In the case of the femoral sheath, the initial elevation, dissection, and division expose the front wall of the common femoral artery with the loose periarterial tissue immediately surrounding it. The incision in the femoral sheath can then be rapidly extended both proximally and distally to expose the common femoral vessel throughout its length.

DISSECTION OF ARTERIES

When arteries are mobilized, the safest plane to dissect is in the plane of Leriche—the periadventitial plane (Fig. 2-10). This plane exists because of the mobility of the arterial wall and the pulsatile nature of flow within the artery itself, and the plane provides safe primary access to every blood vessel. The use of forceps and scissors as shown in the figure allows the precise identification of the periadventitial plane. On occasion, however, secondary planes of dissection, which are inherently more dangerous, must be used because of a previous attempt at mobilization of an artery, the inflammatory component of the disease process in the arterial wall, or periarterial

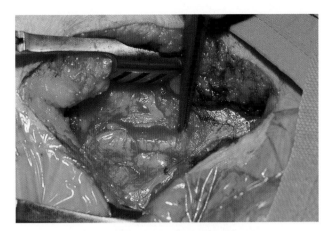

Figure 2-10. Arterial mobilization in the plane of Leriche.

fibrosis from healing or resolving hematoma, particularly after angiography. It should be noted that previously mobilized arteries attempt to regenerate the plane of Leriche, and with the passage of time, the plane becomes better defined. When an artery is occluded, the periadventitial plane is obliterated, and mobilization may have to be performed slightly external to the usual and preferred dissection plane.

We still prefer circumferential mobilization of the vessel because this allows best access to the disease and facilitates external assessment of the disease process (Fig. 2-11). In particular, it allows the determination of endpoint transition from diseased to normal arteries when endarterectomy is the method of treatment of choice.

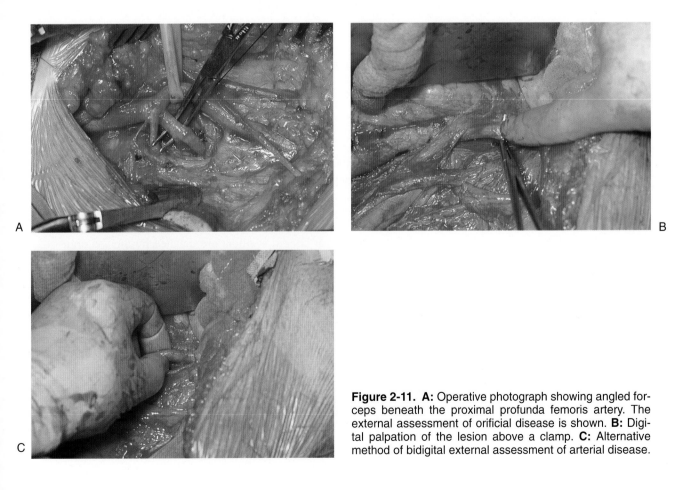

Figure 2-11. A: Operative photograph showing angled forceps beneath the proximal profunda femoris artery. The external assessment of orificial disease is shown. **B:** Digital palpation of the lesion above a clamp. **C:** Alternative method of bidigital external assessment of arterial disease.

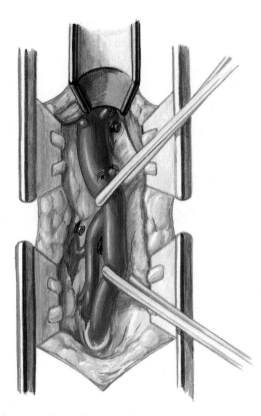

Figure 2-12. Soft plasma tubing slings used to elevate and displace the common femoral bifurcation to visualize the profunda origin. The lateral circumflex iliac vein branches have been divided to further visualize the proximal profunda femoris artery.

In the case of the femoral vessels, however, these are rarely limiting considerations. It is often better to clamp the distal external iliac artery rather than the common femoral artery, as the iliac vessel is predictably less diseased than its femoral continuation. Once a vessel has been mobilized circumferentially, arterial slings are used to provide retraction and, if required, control of an artery (Fig. 2-12). Soft rubber or plastic tubing is the preferred option. These slings permit the arterial segment to be elevated with minimal distortion as any residual loose periarterial tissue is dissected.

The exposure must be designed to display the diseased arterial segment. At a minimum, the exposure allows access to sufficient normal proximal artery for the safe application of the clamps or occluding devices and to minimally diseased distal vessels in general. It is recognized that the amount of artery available and the sites of proximal and distal control of an arterial segment are dictated by the anatomic considerations of the artery in question as well as the extent of the disease (Fig. 2-13).

Ligation of Branches and Tributaries

During the mobilization of arteries and veins, on occasion branches or tributaries will need to be ligated and divided. The correct technique requires that a sufficient length of the branch be mobilized to allow the application of clamps and the secure placement of the ligature.

A common error in the placement of the distal ligature occurs when the vessel has not been mobilized sufficiently and the tie is applied to soft tissue around the vessel. The arterial branch will often "slip away" and not be ligated.

Although one should not leave too long a proximal stump either, leaving too short a distance between the ligature and the clamp results in "tenting" of the vessel with the

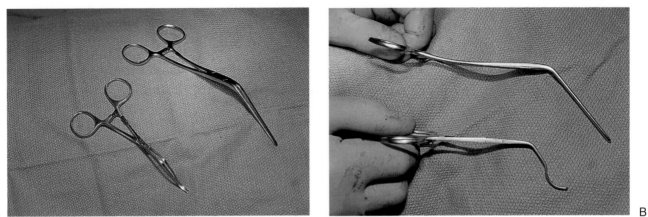

A   B

Figure 2-13. Photograph of arterial clamps (angled Debakey arterial clamp and a profunda clamp) that are employed in these groin procedures.

potential for narrowing the vessel, inducing thrombosis, or losing the ligature with resultant hemorrhage.

Exposure of the Common Femoral Artery and Its Branches

Earlier in the chapter we described the initial skin incision and development of the superficial route to the front of the femoral sheath (Fig. 2-14). When the roof of the femoral sheath over the artery is incised, the only structures at risk for damage are the femoral branch of the genitofemoral nerve and the branches of the femoral artery

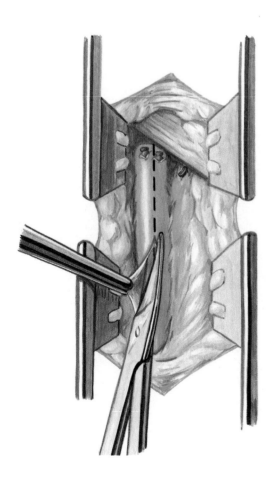

Figure 2-14. Surgeon opening the femoral sheath to expose the underlying femoral artery.

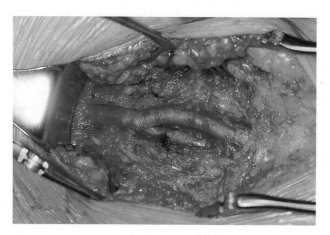

Figure 2-15. Operative photograph showing the common femoral bifurcation exposed with a small tributary ligated adjacent to the profunda femoris artery.

itself. The femoral vein and the branches of the femoral nerve are sequestered away in the other compartments of the femoral sheath and, even after circumferential mobilization of the artery, will be protected. This incision of the femoral sheath can be carried easily up to the inguinal ligament (Fig. 2-15).

Once the inguinal ligament is on display, if an aortofemoral graft is to be placed, the lower one-eighth of the inguinal ligament is divided, or the anterior surface of the femoral artery is separated from it by retraction and elevation of the ligament (Fig. 2-16). The circumflex iliac vein is found coursing across in front of the terminal part of

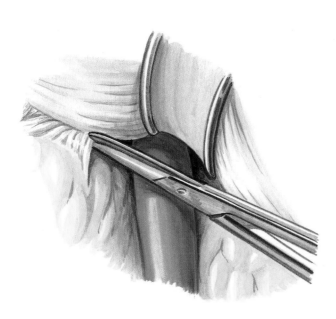

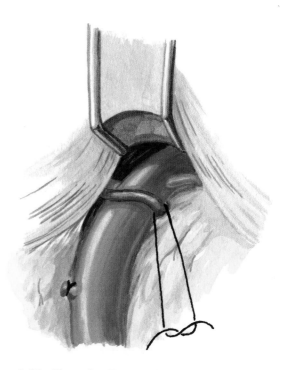

Figure 2-16. Lateral mobilization of the inguinal region to facilitate elevating the inguinal ligament for proximal exposure of the external iliac–common femoral artery junction.

Figure 2-17. Circumflex iliac vein (vein of sorrow) crossing the distal external iliac artery above the level of the inguinal ligament.

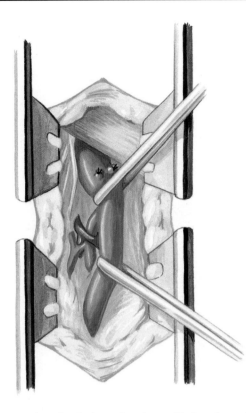

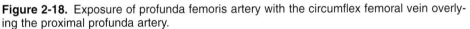

Figure 2-18. Exposure of profunda femoris artery with the circumflex femoral vein overlying the proximal profunda artery.

the external iliac artery. This can be controlled with long straight clamps and ligation of the vessel (Fig. 2-17).

This dissection is the beginning of the retroperitoneal tunnel from the groin exposure. Once the vein has been mobilized safely and its divided ends are ligated, the tunnel is developed easily on the lateral aspect of the external iliac artery, where it abuts on the iliac fascia covering the psoas major muscle. This placement of the tunnel not only is the easiest one but also represents the safest anatomic route, as it avoids a substantial amount of the lymphatics. Careful attention to detail, with the finger being at all times in contact with the outer surface of the iliac artery, ensures that penetration of the peritoneum does not occur.

Inferiorly, the superficial femoral artery can be mobilized by continuation distally of the incision of the femoral sheath and the periadventitial tissue. The first 5 cm or more of superficial femoral artery can be easily dissected and mobilized circumferentially. Once the artery has disappeared behind the sartorius muscle, sharp dissection of the medial border of the sartorius muscle and lateral retraction of the muscle belly unroofs the subsartorial canal. The superficial femoral artery can be dissected for an extended distance.

This mobilization of the superficial femoral artery is also required to facilitate exposure of the profunda femoris vessel (Fig. 2-18). Once a length of superficial femoral artery has been exposed and mobilized, the origin of the profunda femoris is identified at the bifurcation. The origin of the profunda artery is dissected free of its investing periadventitial tissue. The first structure that dissection encounters is the circumflex femoral vein. This vein must be divided and suture ligated to permit access to

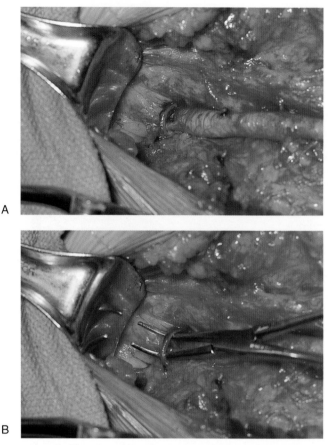

Figure 2-19. Operative photographs. **A:** The circumflex iliac vein crossing the distal external iliac artery. **B:** The clamp beneath the vein, opened in preparation for clamping and ligating the structure.

the anterior surface of the profunda femoris artery (Fig. 2-19). Once that has been done, the profunda trunk can be exposed to its distal third, where it pierces adductor magnus, by mobilization of the lateral margin of adductor longus muscle and medial retention of that muscle belly. The lateral margin of adductor longus is dissected free and retracted medially to expose the trunk of the profunda femoris artery (Fig. 2-20). The continuation distally of the groin dissection into the thigh is facilitated by mobilization and retention of the muscle bellies that cover and protect these important arteries as they course through the musculature of the thigh (Fig. 2-21).

During femoropopliteal or femorodistal reconstructions, a tunnel must be formed from the femoral triangle and carried more distally into the leg. Three options are available: subcutaneous, subfascial, or the more anatomic placement of the tunnel graft in the subsartorial canal. We regard anatomic placement of the tunnel as the best option. It is the safest and conforms best to our definition of exposure. It is also the most technically difficult to create, not in its upper extent but in the area of adductor hiatus in some patients. However, the advantages of following the natural pathway, with viable muscle tissue surrounding the graft and the good control of fluid and blood accumulations from there being no dead space, far outweigh these potential technical difficulties.

If the subsartorial tunnel is begun from the groin exposure, the apex of the femoral triangle is widened, and a finger is inserted on the anterolateral aspect of the superficial femoral artery. The dissecting finger is advanced, and the fingernail's contact with the arterial wall is maintained. If required, a rigid tunneling device can be used to

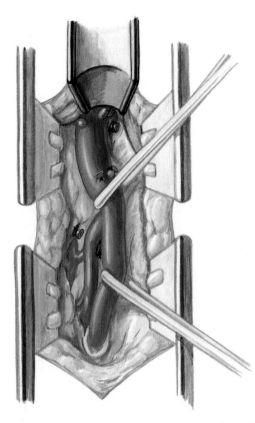

Figure 2-20. Soft plasma tubing slings used to elevate and displace the common femoral bifurcation to visualize the profunda origin. The lateral circumflex iliac vein branches have been divided to further visualize the proximal clip under the femoris artery.

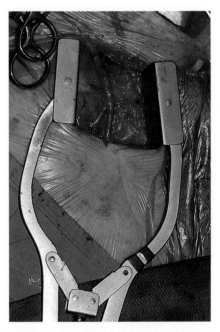

Figure 2-21. Operative photograph of groin exposure held by mechanical retractor. Note the mobilized external iliac artery above and the proximal superficial femoral artery below.

broaden the tunnel. Maintenance of the position behind sartorius below the quite strong musculofascial roof of the canal and anterolateral to the artery avoids any potential injury to nervous or venous structures within the canal. Damage to the saphenous nerve within the canal is a source of some morbidity to patients, and careful attention to the tunneling avoids that problem.

If necessary, the tunnel can be created subfascially by beginning underneath the fascia lata and extending across the sartorius into the groove between sartorius and gracilis and entering the popliteal space between sartorius and gracilis. This offers the best and least risky route of the tunnel in the subfascial space. Although some surgeons prefer to place the tunnel using the subcutaneous space, and particularly the site of harvest of the long saphenous vein, this is our least preferred option.

At the completion of the mobilization, it has become our practice to review critically the wound and its components, including the routes to the artery and any tunnels so formed. We do this before performing the index operation and before the heparin has been given. At that time, any injury to lymph nodes or areas of bleeding that have been unrecognized previously are attended to with excision of the node, diathermy of small bleeding points, and ligature of any obvious vascular or lymphatic channels. We believe that at the completion of the vascular exposure, if the index procedure in that anatomic area is not to proceed immediately, and when complete retraction and retention are not required for access, the retraction and retention should be released to prevent unnecessary pressure on the wounds.

RESTORATION

The restoration of the groin wound is dependent on the wound engineering that has created the exposure. One is also required to follow the hierarchy of healing priorities, as in any operative vascular intervention, in order to provide the optimum environment for the vascular wound to heal. The vascular wound itself requires coverage with viable tissue; thus, the perivascular structures must be coapted. The route of access to the vessel and the skin must be returned to as near normal in conformation as possible. In the previously unoperated groin, the tissue planes that hold suture material well include the femoral sheath, the fascia lata, the membranous layer of the superficial fascia, and the immediate subcuticular tissue. Thus, it is possible to coapt four layers without tension in most patients having their groins opened (Fig. 2-22).

Although classical teaching has been that the femoral sheath should not be closed over implanted grafts because of a concern about compression, it has become our practice to do so. Femoral sheath is a resilient structure; it holds sutures well and is capable of bringing healthy, well-vascularized tissue in direct contact with the arterial wound. Coaptation of the sheath excludes the layers of fatty and lymphatic-rich tissue above which are potential sources of contaminated or sterile fluid accumulation. Thus, we attempt to ensure a tension-free closure of the femoral sheath in all cases of primary arterial repair and in all cases where it is technically possible when a graft is in position. This can be accomplished as a separate layer.

Frequently we use a somewhat different technique. We begin a suture at the level of the inguinal ligament and, sewing inferiorly, close the femoral sheath. The suture is brought back in the layer of the fascia lata, providing a secure fascial closure and totally excluding the superficial lymph nodes from any capacity to leak onto the arterial repair. When the membranous layer of superficial fascia is closed, careful attention should be given to the alignment of the skin wound during the closure. Appropriate corrective action should be taken by taking slightly larger bites on one side or other during the closure of that layer to ensure that the skin is aligned and evenly spaced on both sides of the wound. If the membranous layer of superficial fascia is closed carefully, a very fine subcuticular layer ensures tension-free coaption of the skin. Thus, the principles we try to embody are a firm closure over the

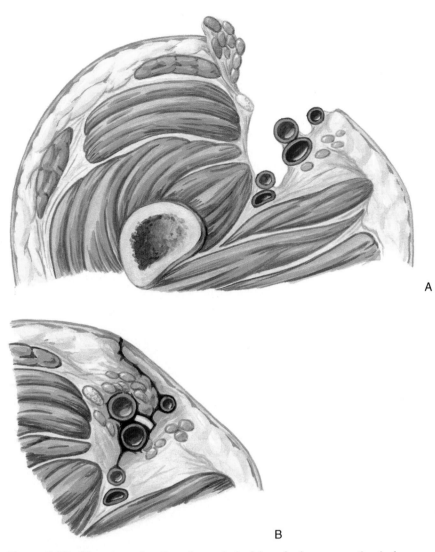

A

B

Figure 2-22. Steps in restoration of a groin incision. **A:** A cross section before wound closure. **B:** Placement of a drain adjacent to the vessels and a layered approximation of the wound to eliminate dead space.

arterial wound and repair, coaption of the routes of access, and tension-free approximation of the skin.

As stated earlier, if lymph nodes are damaged during the exposure, these are excised. If there is accumulation of fluid consistently in the wound with no obvious source, a drain is placed in the layers between the fascia lata and membranous layer of the superficial fascia to ensure obliteration of dead space and removal of any accumulated fluid. The drains are brought out through a separate stab incision, conforming to our practice and beliefs in exposure with a separate exit wound and particular route of access to achieve the specific purpose of the suction drain.

THE REOPERATIVE GROIN

A common phenomenon for us has been the necessity to reoperate in a groin that has been opened either to repair some complication of a previously placed aortofemoral or femoral–popliteal graft or to originate a more distally seeking graft after a proximal reconstruction.

Depending on its pathology, the reoperative groin may be technically challenging, but on most occasions the reexploration is tedious. Our experience has led us to the belief that the most important principle to be adopted is to try and convert the previously scarred operative field to as near "primary operative condition by the end of the procedure as is possible." This implies the redevelopment of the access route that the original surgeon took to the vessel, the identification and mobilization of the vessels, and, when it is safe to do so, excision of as much of the previously laid down scar tissue as is practical before closure restoration. It is surprising how narrow the fibrous scarred zone is in reoperated groins that were handled diligently, left dry, and in which there were no healing complications. Groins where there was previous superficial infection or lymphocoeles frequently have widely dispersed areas of scar and anomalous healing, which make the goal of attainment of normal restoration more difficult.

The patient is positioned similarly to the position used in the primary operation; the original skin scar is incised, and the scar tissue is followed so that the original surgeon's steps are faithfully retraced. In the dense scar of the reoperative wound, we sometimes use sharp-pointed tenotomy scissors to establish and continue appropriate paths to the vessels. The fine handles and small cutting area of the blades allow the successful performance of the periarterial dissection of previously mobilized arteries with minimal risk of arterial injury.

Once the level of the reconstituted femoral sheath has been attained, it is frequently easier to dissect more proximally and mobilize and trace a previous aortofemoral graft to the femoral artery. Alternatively, it may be desirable to proceed more distally and find previously undissected vessels and mobilize these circumferentially. The aims of both these maneuvers is the same: to ensure that the vascular mobilization is carried out in the true periadvential plane, thereby minimizing the risks to the artery itself and to the surrounding structures.

Vessels that are patent even though they have been previously mobilized attempt to regenerate the plane of Leriche, and it is easier to identify this reformed plane if a previously undissected adjacent artery is mobilized and the depth for the proper dissection plane is established. A previously implanted graft, once it has been mobilized from its perigraft capsule, will also lead the surgeon to the correct dissection plane.

Thus, in general, the plan for the previously operated groin is to carefully retrace the surgeon's footsteps, as this is safe through a preestablished route of access. Then it is possible to establish the appropriate level of dissection and to remobilize the arteries circumferentially as required. The appropriate excision of scar tissue, and replacement of this with well-vascularized normal tissue, is the goal for us prior to and during restoration which should follow the previously described pattern. Suction drainage is mandatory.

LATERAL APPROACH TO THE BRANCHES OF THE FEMORAL ARTERY

On occasion, the pathology in the groin, such as infection within the femoral triangle, precludes or demands an alternative route of access to the femoral vessels. Again, the anatomy of the region is brought into play.

The incision is made beginning two to three inches below the anterior superior iliac spine and along the lateral margin of the sartorius. This incision is deepened, the lateral margin of sartorius elevated, and a clean dissection plane behind sartorius is used to identify the superficial femoral and profunda femoris arteries. In this exposure the muscle belly of sartorius is retained medially, and if required, the medial side of adductor longus is mobilized and retained laterally to expose the mid third of the profunda femoris artery.

Thus, the femoral vessels can be approached through clean tissue planes to provide suitable access for an extra anatomic bypass in a clean exposure excluding an area of contamination or frank sepsis. Conceptually, this accords with our principles of exposure and allows for precise restoration of anatomy at the completion of the vascular procedure.

3
Neck

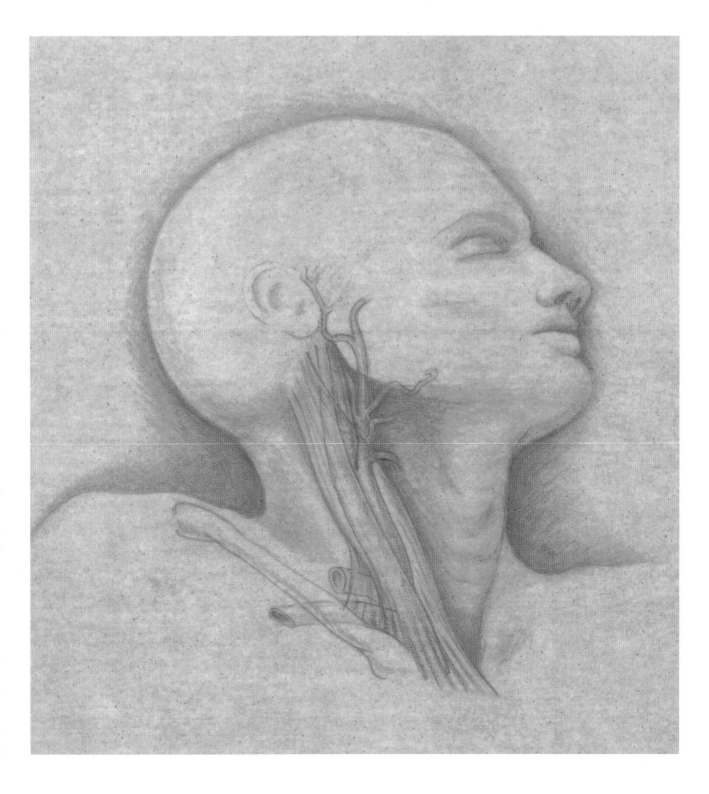

In this chapter we consider the exposures of the cervical portions of the common carotid artery and its major branches.

SURGICAL ANATOMY

The muscular key to the neck is the sternocleidomastoid muscle, which divides the neck into the two primary regions, the anterior and posterior triangles, and overlies and protects the blood supply to and the venous drainage from the brain. If the sternocleidomastoid muscle is removed, the major neurovascular bundles of the neck are visualized, cradled by the deep musculature of the neck (Fig. 3-2).

The next key to adept surgical exposure of the vessels within the neck is to understand the anatomy of the internal jugular vein and to be able to mobilize it.

The sternocleidomastoid muscle is a prominent landmark in the neck of most humans. It arises from two heads: a sternal head, which is a tendinous origin, and a more fleshy clavicular head from the superior border and anterior surface of the middle third of the clavicle. The two heads are separated by a small triangular space with the sternal head passing obliquely and the clavicular head passing almost directly cephalad to form a strong muscular belly, which then inserts into the lateral surface of the mastoid process and to the adjoining superior nuchal line of the occipital bone.

The sternocleidomastoid muscle is surrounded by the deep cervical fascia, which, after covering the roof of the posterior triangle, splits to enclose the sternocleidomastoid muscle and rejoins at the anterior border of that muscle to form a definite single lamina. The lamina covers the anterior triangle of the neck and extends to the median plane of the neck. This fascia has several condensations in it including the stylomandibular ligament. Where the fascia splits to enclose the parotid gland, it assumes the name of that gland.

Superficial to the sternocleidomastoid muscle is the platysma, a broad sheet of thin muscle arising from the fascia covering the upper parts of pectoralis major and deltoid and inserted into the skin and subcutaneous tissue of the lower part of the face and neck. The external jugular vein, which descends across the sternocleidomastoid under the cover of platysma muscle from the angle of the mandible to approximately the

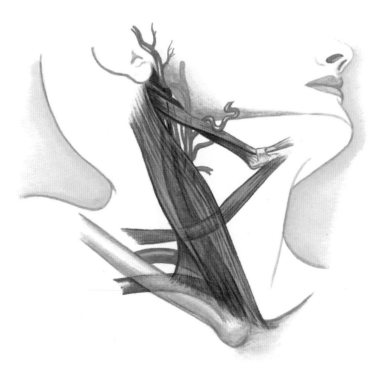

Figure 3-2. Side of neck and selected anatomy.

middle of the clavicle, is a superficial relation. The deep surface of the muscle lies on the strap muscles and the omohyoid muscle, the anterior jugular vein, and the carotid sheath. It has many neural relationships including the cervical plexus, the upper part of the brachial plexus, and the phrenic nerve. The posterior part of the muscle is related to the splenius capitis, levator scapulae, and the scalene muscles. The sternocleidomastoid is supplied by the accessory nerve and by parts of the second and third cervical nerves. If the sternocleidomastoid muscle, the investing fascia, and the lymph nodes of the deep cervical chain are removed by dissection, the vasculature of the neck can be divided into three parts by two crossing muscle bellies, the postposterior belly of digastric and the inferior belly of omohyoid. Our discussion in this chapter concentrates mainly on the portions of the vessels above the omohyoid muscle (Figs. 3-3 and 3-4).

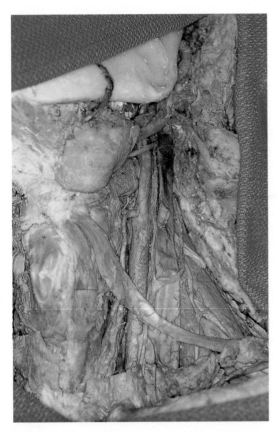

Figure 3-3. Cadaver dissection showing carotid artery and related anatomic structures.

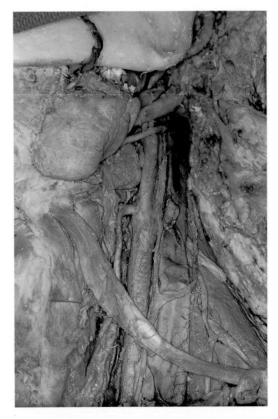

Figure 3-4. Cadaver dissection showing close-up view of carotid bifurcation and crossing omohyoid muscle.

The internal jugular vein begins at the base of the skull, where it emerges through the jugular foramen as a direct continuation of the sigmoid sinus. The jugular bulb is the name applied to the first part of the jugular vein, which is slightly dilated. The vein runs downward through the neck within the carotid sheath and ends behind the sternal end of the clavicle, where it unites with the subclavian vein to form the brachio-cephalic vein. The internal jugular vein is overlapped by the upper part and covered by the lower part of the sternocleidomastoid and the two crossing muscles. Above the digastric muscle, it is covered by the parotid gland. The styloid process and the accessory nerve, on its path to the sternocleidomastoid muscle, cross superficial to it. Posteriorly the internal jugular vein rests on, in descending order, levator scapulae, scalenus medius, the cervical plexus, and then on the scalenus anterior and the phrenic nerve. On the left side an important posterior relation is the thoracic duct as it winds its way around to seek entry into the junction of the internal jugular and subclavian veins. On the medial side the vein is related to the internal and common carotid arteries, also lying within the carotid sheath, with the vagus nerve between the vein and the arteries but on a plane that is posterior to the vessels. The important cervical tributaries include the veins of the tongue and pharynx, the occipital and common facial veins, and the superior thyroid vein. This latter begins in the substance of the thyroid gland, accompanies the superior thyroid artery, and ends in the internal jugular vein.

The common facial vein is a very important landmark in the neck. Below and in front of the angle of the mandible, a large retromandibular vein joins it, and the vein crosses the lingual artery, the 12th nerve, and both the external and internal carotid arteries to enter the internal jugular vein at about the level of the greater horn of the hyoid bone. It is important as a landmark because it usually overlies the bifurcation of the carotid artery.

The common carotid artery has a different origin on each side of the neck. The right begins at the bifurcation of the brachiocephalic artery, whereas the left arises from the arch of the aorta itself, behind and to the left of the brachiocephalic trunk. The cervical portions of the common carotid arteries have an almost identical course with the exception that, because of their different origins, the left common carotid is more deeply placed in the neck behind the anterior border of the sternocleidomastoid than its counterpart on the right.

The common carotid artery typically passes without a branch to about the level of the thyroid cartilage, where it divides into the internal carotid and external carotid vessels. The proximal part of the internal carotid artery is dilated and is called the carotid bulb. The carotid sinus baroreceptor is within the bulb, and the carotid body, a chemoreceptor, lies in close relation to its bifurcation and between the internal and external carotid. The superior and lateral relations are covered by knowledge of the anatomy of the jugular vein with an important addition. Just above the bifurcation, the internal and external carotid arteries are crossed by the 12th nerve where it curves forward around the sternocleidomastoid branch. This nerve is an immediate relation of the jugular vein and of both branches of the carotid artery.

Posteriorly the common carotid artery is separated from the transverse processes of the cervical vertebrae by longus colli and longus capitis muscles, the origin of scalenus anterior muscle, and the sympathetic trunk. Its medial relations include the esophagus, trachea, inferior thyroid artery, and recurrent laryngeal nerves, and higher in the neck the larynx and pharynx are immediate medial relations of the vessel.

The internal carotid artery is divided into four parts, of which we describe only the cervical. This is the continuation of the common carotid artery, and it usually begins at the upper border of the thyroid cartilage. Posteriorly the vessel rests on longus capitis with the superior cervical sympathetic ganglion between it and the muscle. The superior laryngeal nerve crosses obliquely behind it. The internal carotid is directly related to the wall of the pharynx with only some fat and the pharyngeal veins between the two. Anterolaterally the internal carotid artery is covered by the sternocleidomastoid muscle and the digastric muscle, which crosses it. Below the digastric muscle, the internal carotid artery is related to the hypoglossal nerve and the ansa cervicalis. The landmark that identifies the bifurcation is the junction of the common facial vein with the internal jugular vein. Above the digastric muscle, the styloid process and styloglossus complex intervene between the internal and external carotid arteries, as do the glossopharyngeal nerve, some branches of the vagus, and the deep lobe of the parotid gland. As the artery approaches the base of the skull, the ninth, tenth, 11th, and 12th cranial nerves lie between the internal carotid artery and the internal jugular vein, which, by that stage, has assumed a position posterior to the artery. The internal carotid artery enters the skull through the foramen lacerum in the temporal bone.

The external carotid artery is an artery of supply to the muscles and viscera of the face and neck. Accordingly, its main trunk is short, and it promptly breaks into its branches—the superior thyroid, ascending pharyngeal, lingual, fascial, occipital, posterior auricular, and maxillary—before continuing as the superficial temporal artery. The superior thyroid is an important vessel as it arises from the front of the external carotid artery almost at the bifurcation, and in a number of patients it arises from the common carotid artery itself. The sternocleidomastoid branch of the occipital artery is the vascular leash around which the hypoglossal nerve turns forward on its journey to supply the tongue.

The carotid sheath is a condensation of the cervical fascia in which the common and internal carotid arteries, the jugular vein and vagus nerve, as well as the ansa cervicalis are contained. It is a definite layer easily identified where it is related to the arteries, but because of the great distensibility of the internal jugular vein, the fascia is considerably thinned out over that structure.

POSITIONING OF THE PATIENT

The patient should be positioned comfortably on the operating table, and after induction of anesthesia, the table should be broken so that both the head and feet are somewhat elevated (semi-Fowler's position) (Fig. 3-5). The neck is then hyperextended by positioning a sandbag beneath the shoulders and a ring under the head, and the headpiece of the table is lowered. The face is turned away from the side being operated on. The final position should ensure that the neck is flat but above the level of the heart to ensure that the internal jugular vein remains decompressed throughout the operative procedure.

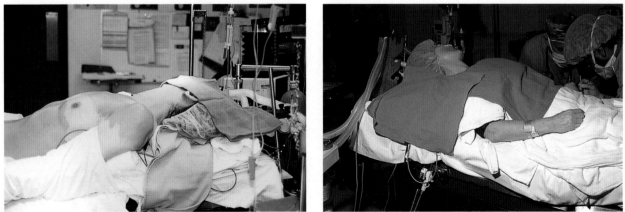

Figure 3-5. A: Position of patient with head rotated to opposite side and patient in semi-Fowler's position. **B:** Positioning for exposure of lateral neck.

EXPOSURE OF THE CAROTID BIFURCATION

The carotid bifurcation may be exposed through either a skin crease incision placed over the bifurcation or by a more vertically placed but still oblique incision following the anterior border of the sternocleidomastoid (Fig. 3-6) Both of these incisions give good access to the bifurcation and to the internal and external carotid arteries. The transverse incision may be limiting when substantial access is required to the proximal common carotid artery. A greater length of common carotid artery can be mobilized through the anterior border of the sternocleidomastoid incision, which may be extended caudally as required.

The skin is divided by a sharp scalpel with the blade held at right angles to the skin. The platysma muscle is divided in the same line as the skin incision. When the platysma is divided, the skin wound will spring apart slightly. If the transverse incision has been used, the great auricular nerve will be visualized at the most posterior part of the incision. Great care is taken to avoid damage to this nerve because, if it is damaged, there is anesthesia of the ear and adjacent skin that has proven to be irritating to all patients who have had this injury. In all patients having an exposure of the carotid bifurcation, some sensory fibers of the cervical plexus are divided, and this is manifest postoperatively by minor areas of cutaneous anesthesia or hypesthesia in the neck, which usually recover.

If the transverse incision is used, subplatysmal flaps are created by sharp dissection in the plane on the surface of the fascia covering the sternocleidomastoid muscle. This plane is developed superiorly as far as necessary to mobilize the anterior border of the sternocleidomastoid and is then dissected inferiorly, effectively converting the transverse incision into a longitudinal exposure.

After the creation of these flaps, or if the oblique incision has been used, the anterior border of the sternocleidomastoid muscle is identified, and the investing layer of the deep cervical fascia is incised immediately in front of this border. The dissection is carried cephalad and caudad in order to mobilize the anterior border and posterior surface of the muscle to allow for visualization of the neurovascular bundle and lateral retention of the muscle out of the field after retraction has been established. The dissection and reflection of the sternocleidomastoid expose the internal jugular vein through the thinned-out carotid sheath.

As indicated previously, the second key to safe and efficient mobilization of the carotid arteries is a thorough mobilization of the internal jugular vein (Fig. 3-7). The vein should be mobilized initially from the sheath along the anteromedial border of the vein by making a vertical incision in the sheath. The dissection is then carried inferi-

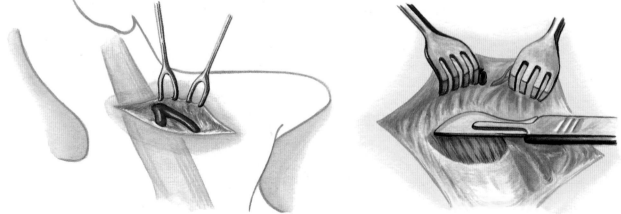

A   B

Figure 3-6. Transverse incision centered over carotid bifurcation area **(A)** and subplatysmal flap created **(B)**.

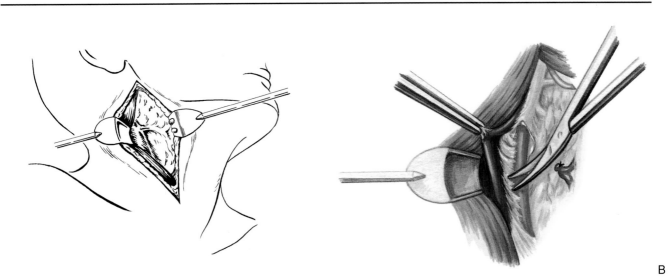

A

B

Figure 3-7. Dissection separating the carotid artery from its attachments to the adjacent jugular vein.

orly to the omohyoid muscle. Superiorly the dissection is carried as far as necessary to ensure adequate mobilization of disease-free internal carotid artery. Adhering to this anterior border of the jugular vein carries the dissection posterior to the 12th nerve by allowing a very clear demonstration of the path of the descendens hypoglossi in the anterior lamella of the carotid sheath.

The level of the carotid bifurcation is marked by the entry of the common facial vein into the internal jugular vein. The common facial vein is mobilized and divided between clamps. Both ends of the divided vein are suture ligated. Further mobilization of the internal jugular vein then proceeds cephalad with division of any further small tributaries that cause annoying bleeding if injured inadvertently. The jugulo-digastric lymph node mass is identified and displaced anteromedially, but if it is very bulky and obscuring access, it should be resected (Fig. 3-8). Mobilization of the internal jugular vein is carried cephalad at least as far as the posterior belly of the digastric.

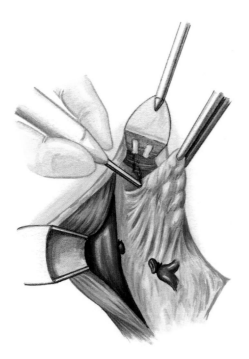

Figure 3-8. Removal of jugular digastric node and adjacent lymphatics.

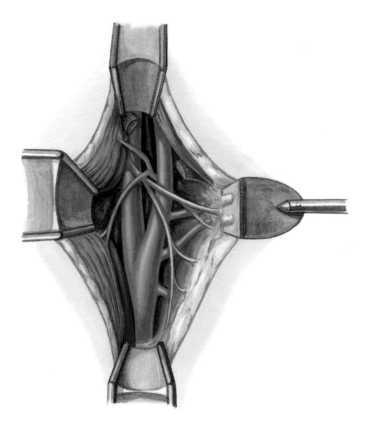

Figure 3-9. Completely mobilized common carotid artery and bifurcation branches.

At the completion of this dissection, the sternocleidomastoid muscle and the jugular vein can be retained posterolaterally by self-retaining retractors to expose the common carotid bifurcation and internal and external carotid vessels (Fig. 3-9). No attempt is made to mobilize the vagus nerve, which usually can be seen in the base of the dissection between the carotid and internal jugular vein. In addition to avoiding dissecting the nerve, great care is taken when placing the retractors to hold the jugular and sternocleidomastoid out of the operative field because the vagus nerve may be damaged during the placement of these instruments at this stage of the procedure (Fig. 3-10).

We expose the carotid artery by an incision into the carotid sheath behind the descendens hypoglossi, thus preserving a considerable portion of the carotid sheath anterior to the vagus. On occasions the course of the vagus nerve is aberrant. This occurs more commonly on the right side than the left, and the vagus occupies a position anterior in the areolar tissue of the sheath. This is occasionally associated with a direct rather than a recurrent laryngeal nerve. In reoperative surgery of this region, particularly if the vagus has been dissected in any way, it is drawn up into the healing ridge around the carotid artery and may present quite anteriorly of the carotid artery. The carotid artery is approached from the posterolateral aspect by scissors and forceps dissection. The carotid sheath is incised behind the decendens hypoglossi, and great care is taken to identify and remain in the true periadventitial plane. Appropriate dissection during mobilization of the carotid arteries facilitates closure of the vascular wound after the completion of any procedure. The dissection proceeds with circumferential mobilization of the common carotid artery, which is then carried cephalad on the internal carotid artery behind the decendens hypoglossi nerve. The sternocleidomastoid branch of the occipital artery and its accompanying vein are identified and ligated. This allows the hypoglossal nerve to move forward to a more anterior position. The division of this bundle, which often marks the end of the carotid bulb, allows the surgeon access to the very fine areolar tissue that surrounds the more distal internal

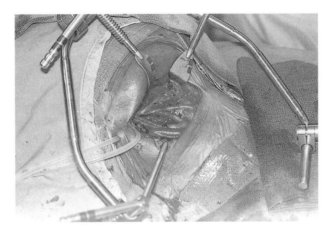

Figure 3-10. Operative photograph showing self-retaining table-mounted retractor system providing exposure for the mobilized carotid bifurcation.

cervical carotid artery. Dissection then proceeds smoothly until sufficient length of internal carotid has been mobilized.

The external carotid artery is mobilized by dissecting the anteromedial border of the bifurcation and extending that incision along the external carotid. The vessel is always mobilized beyond its first bifurcation to encompass the extent of disease.

The final part of this exposure involves mobilizing the carotid bulb itself. Slings of plastic or rubber tubing are placed around the mobilized common, internal, and external carotid arteries. These are used as retractors to gently elevate the vessels, thus facilitating the dissection of the patient away from the bulb rather than dissecting the bulb from the patient. When the carotid bulb is mobilized, great care is again taken to remain in the true periadventitial plane, as this protects the superior laryngeal nerve, which crosses behind the bulb to reach its anatomic relationship with the superior laryngeal artery. Dissection in that plane is absolutely vital to preserve the arterial wall and allow accurate repair during restoration.

The final step is to elevate and dissect the posterior surface of the bulb to completely free the bifurcation. This allows the rotation required to prepare the artery for arteriotomy (Fig. 3-11).

In summary, the exposure of the carotid artery follows clear anatomic routes and fulfills the principles we have adopted. As in all exposures, before any anticoagulants are administered, the wound is carefully examined for any bleeding sites or potential lymph leaks. Any nonviable tissue or damaged lymph nodes are excised at this stage.

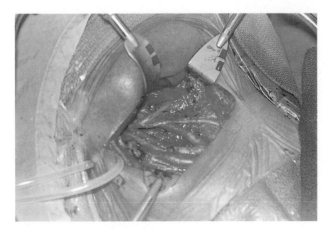

Figure 3-11. Operative photograph showing in close-up the details of the carotid bifurcation and related anatomy.

RESTORATION

The neck is rich in arterial and venous supply, and the arterial repair is easily covered with viable tissue. However, there is potential for fluid accumulation, and the exposure described creates potential dead space, particularly when the jugular–digastric lymph node mass is excised. Thus, we have adopted the practice of routinely draining the neck, using closed-system suction drains, after ensuring that the wound and routes of access to the carotid are completely dry (Fig. 3-12). The drain is brought out

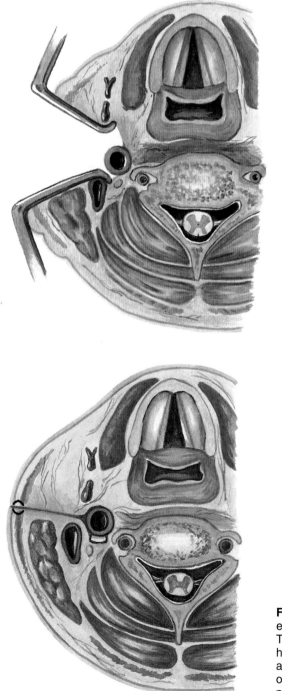

A

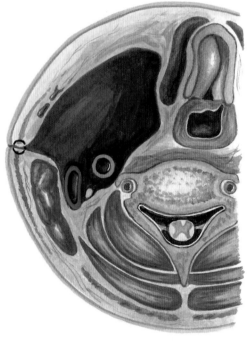

B

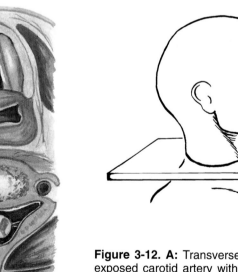

C

Figure 3-12. A: Transverse section showing the exposed carotid artery with wound retraction. **B:** Transverse view of closed wound with a large hematoma surrounding the carotid and displacing and compromising the airway. **C:** Transverse view of neck with a closed wound. Drains have been placed adjacent to the carotid artery.

through a separate trochar wound and is placed deep to the investing fascia. The platysma is closed using absorbable suture material, and care is taken in that closure to ensure that the skin wound is not distorted. The skin edges are approximated.

This closure illustrates the principles of preserving the carotid sheath to allow it to fall back and cover the arterial wound, of obliterating dead space, and of removing fluid accumulation by closed suction drainage for 24 hours. Furthermore, the restoration makes use of a layer that holds the sutures well to reposition the other structures, restoring as near normal anatomic arrangement as practical.

UPPER CERVICAL INTERNAL CAROTID ARTERY

Occasionally, because of disease, trauma, or aneurysm, access is required to the segment of the internal carotid artery above the digastric muscle. When this is required, further cephalad dissection is needed to expose the artery to the base of the skull. It is evident from the description of the surgical anatomy in the early part of this chapter that cranial nerves eight, nine, ten, 11, and 12 are at risk in any dissection of that part of the internal carotid artery. In the past, mandibular division was used to reach the vessels that were situated high in the neck. However, in recent times we have learned other ways to approach this more inaccessible part of the internal carotid (Figs. 3-13 and 3-14).

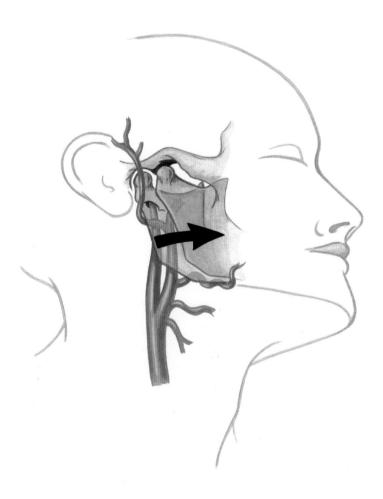

Figure 3-13. Mandible displaced anteriorly, creating an enlarged space behind the ramus of the mandible.

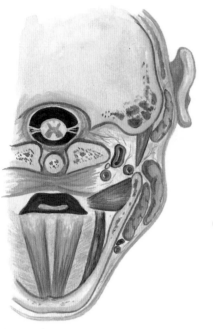
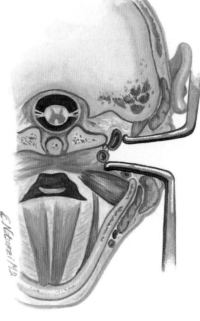
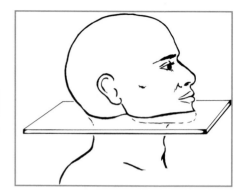

A,B

Figure 3-14. Transverse view of upper neck. **A:** normal anatomy. **B:** the space developed by forward displacement of the mandible. The space created is held in place by wound retractors.

All patients with high carotid lesions should have nasotracheal rather than orotracheal intubation (Fig. 3-15). Removing the endotracheal tube from the mouth allows the jaw to be pronated much further and opens the gap between the ascending ramus of the mandible and the anterior border of the sternocleidomastoid by ~1 to 1.5 cm. In elderly patients with lax temporal mandibular joint ligaments, the jaw is pronated by applying traction to forcibly subluxate the jaw. In those in whom insufficient space would be generated by this maneuver, we now dislocate the jaw at the temporomandibular joint by downward and forward traction. The jaw moves forward, facilitating access to the most distal portions of the internal carotid artery. The incision should be made along the anterior border of the sternocleidomastoid muscle and carried higher than would normally be the case for a bifurcation mobilization. The bifurcation and proximal internal carotid artery should be mobilized, the digastric muscle

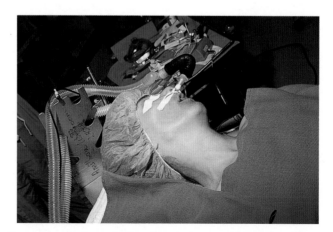

Figure 3-15. Operative photograph showing patient positioned for carotid exposure with nasal intubation.

brought in view, and the posterior belly divided and, if necessary, resected to provide sufficient access. Above the digastric muscle, the structures that lie between the internal and external carotid arteries, particularly the muscles arising from the styloid process, may require division. Likewise, the deep part of the parotid gland will require some mobilization to facilitate the exposure. Careful scissors and forceps dissection then allows extensile exposure of the carotid to the base of the skull.

CERVICAL COMMON CAROTID ARTERY

The cervical component of the common carotid artery above the base of the neck is best approached through an incision along the anterior border of the sternocleidomastoid muscle, and the same technique is used as was described for the carotid bifurcation.

Restoration for both exposures involves closed suction drainage and accurate closure of the platysma with skin approximation.

4

Base of the Neck

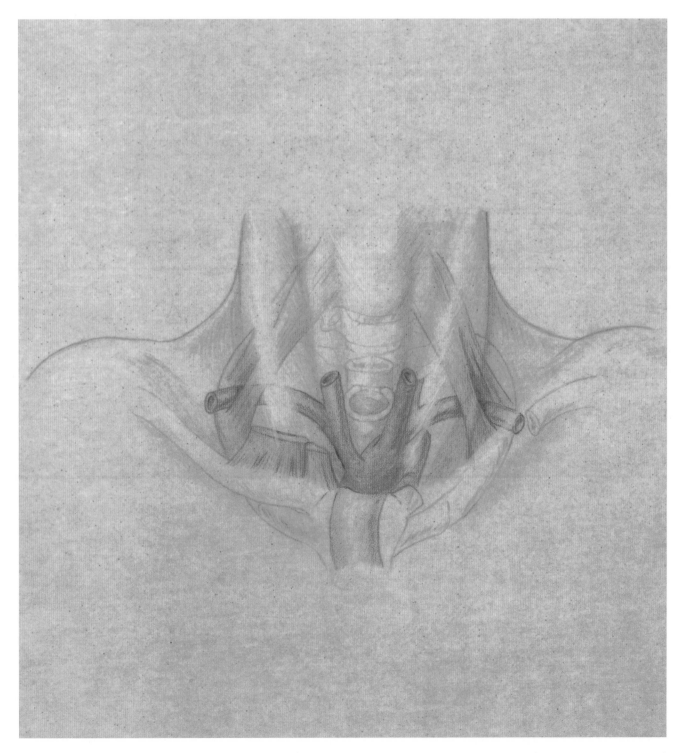

In this chapter we deal with the exposures at the base of the neck. We describe the techniques used to visualize and display not only the vessels but also the major nerves of the region, and we describe an exposure of the first thoracic rib.

SURGICAL ANATOMY

The base of the neck is an area of complex anatomy (Fig. 4-2). The neck rests on an oval base that slopes from posterior to anterior. This base is composed of the thoracic vertebra posteriorly, the first rib, and the top of the manubrium. The vertebral body intrudes into this oval, and anterior to the vertebral body, the visceral compartment transmits the esophagus and trachea as they pass from the neck into the mediastinum.

In addition to the sloping base, there is a horizontal bony component, the clavicle, which extends from the sternoclavicular joint above the first rib articulation medially to the acromion of the scapula laterally. This bone acts as a brace that holds the shoulder back and allows the arm to swing free of the trunk, but it is a truss as well, transmitting some of the weight of the arm back to the axial skeleton. Between the first rib and the clavicle is a space through which pass the vessels and lymphatics of the upper limb en route through the neck from and to the mediastinum and the major nerves of the upper limb descending from their origin in the cervical spinal cord.

Part of the space between the clavicle and first rib is filled in by a small triangular muscle, the subclavius. This muscle arises from the costochondral junction of the first rib to insert into the middle third of the undersurface of the clavicle.

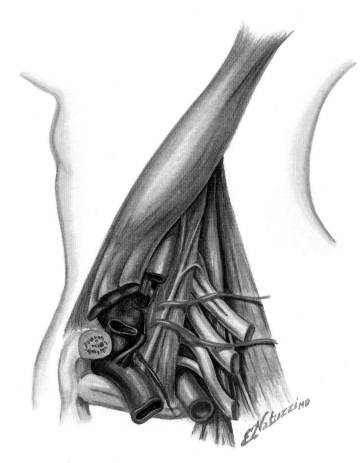

Figure 4-2. Detailed anatomy at the base of the anterolateral neck.

For surgical exposures of neurovascular structures in the root of the neck, the key muscular structures are the lateral vertebral muscles—the scalenus anterior and the scalenus medius. The scalenus posterior is a small, usually insignificant muscle hidden behind the scalenus medius. The structures posterior to scalenus medius—scalenus posterior, the cervical vertebral transverse processes, and the deep muscles of the neck and back—are covered by levator scapulae and wrapped around by trapezius muscle as it comes from the posterior border of the posterior triangle on its way to insert onto the outer third of the clavicle.

The only other posterior muscle of note at the base of the neck is the longus colli. The inferior part arises from the vertebral bodies of T-1 and T-2 and passes upward to attach to the anterior part of the transverse processes of the C-5 and C-6 vertebrae. The middle part of the muscle, which runs vertically, arises from the upper three thoracic and lower three cervical vertebrae.

Scalenus Medius

Scalenus medius is the muscle that provides the key to understanding the anatomy of this part of the neck. Scalenus medius is the largest and longest of the scalene muscles. It arises from the transverse process of the axis and the anterior part of the posterior tubercles of the transverse processes of the lower five cervical vertebrae. On occasion, it also takes origin from the atlas itself. The muscle origins join to form a large muscle belly, which travels obliquely to the outer aspect of the first rib, where it inserts in the upper surface of the first rib, occupying the whole of the space from the groove for the subclavian artery to the tubercle at the angle of the rib.

Thus, at that depth in the neck, we have an almost continuous sheet of muscle—a small amount of levator scapulae above and scalenus medius below—that forms the posterior relationship of the nerves of the cervical and brachial plexus after they emerge from the intervertebral foramina.

Cervical Plexus

The cervical plexus, situated high in the neck, provides the nerve supply of the musculature of the neck and also is the origin of the supraclavicular nerves, which are encountered in any exposure of the base of the neck. These nerves derive from C-3 and C-4 nerve roots, traverse the posterior triangle, pierce the deep fascia, and are distributed as three nerves supplying the lateral, intermediate, and medial components of the skin and subcutaneous tissue overlying the clavicle. The plexus also gives off the descendens cervicalis, which joins with the descendens hypoglossi to form the ansa cervicalis in front of the carotid artery higher in the neck.

Phrenic Nerve

The phrenic nerve is the major motor supply of the diaphragm. Its main origin is from the C-4 cervical nerve, but it receives contributions from C-3 and C-5 as well. The phrenic nerve is formed on the surface of scalenus posterior, at the upper part of the lateral border of scalenus anterior. The nerve passes downward in an almost vertical direction and, because of the origin of scalenus anterior and its site of formation, gains access to the anterior surface of scalenus anterior, which it crosses, and becomes "insolubly wed" to the anterior surface of the muscle, bound there by the prevertebral fascia. After descending on the front of scalenus anterior, the phrenic nerve leaves that muscle on its medial side in the root of the neck. On the right-hand side, it lies lateral to the right brachiocephalic vein and the superior vena cava before attaining the pericardium, where it passes to the diaphragm. The left phrenic nerve, after detaching from scalenus anterior, passes in front of the first part of the left subclavian artery and behind the thoracic duct. As it enters the superior mediastinum, it lies between the left common carotid and subclavian arteries and passes medially and forwards, superficial to the left vagus nerve, above the aortic arch, and behind the left brachiocephalic vein.

Brachial Plexus

The brachial plexus is formed by the ventral rami of C-5, C-6, C-7, and C-8 as well as by a substantial contribution from the first thoracic nerve root. On occasion, there may be a small contribution from the ventral ramus of T-2. These rami are called the roots of the plexus. The C-5 and C-6 roots unite at about the lateral border of scalenus medius to form the upper trunk of the plexus. The C-7 root is the middle trunk, and C-8 and T-1 join to form the lower trunk. The three trunks run downward and laterally, and, at about the level of the clavicle, each trunk splits into an anterior and a posterior division. All three posterior divisions unite to form the posterior cord of the plexus, which lies at first slightly above and then behind the axillary artery. The anterior divisions of the upper and middle trunks unite to form the lateral cord of the plexus, and the anterior division of the lower trunk passes at first behind and then on the medial side of the axillary artery as the medial cord of the plexus.

As is evident from this description, the cords take their names from their relationship to the axillary artery. Only the branches that arise above the clavicle are described here, as they are at risk during some of the exposures. Branches derived from the roots of the plexus supply the scalene muscles and longus colli, and, as indicated previously, the phrenic nerve receives a contribution from C-5.

The nerve to the rhomboid muscles also arises from the roots of C-5 and pierces scalenus medius to run on the deep surface of levator scapulae to the anterior surfaces of the rhomboid muscles. The long thoracic nerve, or the nerve to serratus anterior, arises from the fifth, sixth, and seventh cervical nerve roots. It enters and traverses the substance of scalenus medius to appear on the lateral surface of the muscle, crosses the upper border of scalenus posterior, and continues its descent to the lower border of that muscle, where it lies on the superficial surface serratus anterior supplying the nerves to each of the various interdigitations.

Arteries

As the nerves are descending from their cervical origins, the arteries are coursing upward out of the superior mediastinum to gain access to the neck and upper extremity. On the right side, the brachiocephalic trunk divides at the upper border of the right sternoclavicular joint into the right common carotid and right subclavian arteries. The right common carotid ascends from there as described previously. The left common carotid artery arises directly from the arch of the aorta, behind and to the left of the brachiocephalic trunk, and ascends in the superior mediastinum before traversing the root of the neck to lie in the neurovascular compartment.

The right subclavian artery arises from the brachiocephalic trunk and passes upward and laterally to a point about 2 cm above the clavicle to the medial margin of the scalenus anterior muscle. The artery is covered by the skin, superficial fascia, the clavicular origin of platysma, the anterior supraclavicular nerves, deep fascia, and the clavicular origin of the sternocleidomastoid muscle as well as the strap muscles. It is behind the origin of the right common carotid artery.

As it passes laterally, the subclavian artery is crossed by the vagus nerve, the cardiac branches of that nerve, and by the internal jugular, vertebral, and anterior jugular veins. Inferiorly and posteriorly the artery is related directly to the pleura and apex of the lung, separated from them by the suprapleural membrane (Sibson's fascia). The right recurrent laryngeal nerve passes around the first part of the right subclavian artery.

The first part of the left subclavian artery has a large component within the mediastinum as the artery arises from the arch of the aorta, posterior to and to the left of the left common carotid artery origin. It ascends through the superior mediastinum, through the base of the neck, and arches toward the medial border of scalenus anterior. In the neck the artery is crossed anteriorly by the left phrenic nerve and the terminal part of the thoracic duct.

The second part of each subclavian artery lies behind the scalenus anterior muscle, and behind and below the vessel, the suprapleural membrane, pleura, lung, and the lower trunk of the brachial plexus are immediate relations. Above the second part of each artery are the upper and middle trunks of the plexus. The subclavian vein is below and in front of the artery and separated from it by the insertion of the scalenus anterior muscle.

The third part of the subclavian artery runs downward and laterally from the lateral margin of scalenus anterior toward the outer border of the first rib to become the axillary artery. Here, the artery is easily felt in the supraclavicular fossa.

The subclavian artery has four important branches in the root of the neck—the vertebral artery, the internal mammary artery, the thyrocervical trunk, and the costocervical trunk. The first three of these branches usually take origin close together near the medial border of scalenus anterior and thus, arise from the first part of the vessel.

Vertebral Artery

The vertebral artery arises from the upper and posterior aspect of the first part of the subclavian artery as its first branch. It ascends through the anatomic triangle of the vertebral artery to attain the vertebral foramen in the transverse process of C-6. Its first part is sandwiched between the scalenus anterior and longus colli muscle and behind the common carotid artery. An important posterior relation is the inferior cervical ganglion of the sympathetic trunk and the ventral rami of the seventh and eighth cervical nerves. Once vertebral artery has entered the bony foramina, it passes upward through the vertebral canal to gain entry to the skull.

Internal Mammary Artery

The internal mammary artery arises about 2 cm above the sternal end of the clavicle from the inferior surface of the first part of the subclavian artery, usually opposite the thyrocervical trunk. It descends behind the cartilages of the thorax about 1.5 cm lateral to the sternal edge.

Thyrocervical Trunk

The thyrocervical trunk is a short, wide trunk arising from the front of the first part of the subclavian artery. It divides into three branches—the inferior thyroid, suprascapular, and transverse cervical arteries—all of which are encountered in the dissections required for exposure in this region.

Costocervical Trunk

The costocervical trunk often arises from the second part of the subclavian artery. From there, it arches above the cervical pleura toward the neck of the first rib, where it divides into its two terminal branches.

Thus far, we have built up an arrangement of arteries arising in the mediastinum, traversing the root of the neck, and gaining entry to the arm or ascending through the neck to supply the brain. At the base of the neck, these vessels are joined by the nerves descending through the neck to the viscera or arm. The structures then exit the neck

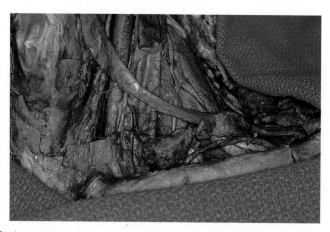

Figure 4-3. Cadaver dissection showing anatomy of the base of the neck.

through the base of the neck or apex of the axilla. All of these structures lie on the muscles previously described (Figs. 4-3 and 4-4).

Muscle Layers

The next layers of muscle protect the nerves and cover the subclavian artery.

Scalenus Anterior

The most important of these muscles is the scalenus anterior, which lies at the side of the neck deep behind the sternocleidomastoid. This muscle arises from the anterior tubercles of the transverse process of the third, fourth, fifth, and sixth cervical vertebrae. It descends at a slightly oblique angle to be inserted into the scalene tubercle on the inner border of the first rib as well as extending onto the upper surface of the rib in front of the groove left by the subclavian artery. In the root of the neck, in front of the muscle, are the clavicle, the subclavius muscle, the sternocleidomastoid muscle, and, on a slightly higher plane, the omohyoid muscle. The lateral portion of the carotid sheath crosses the muscle. Its most important anterior relation, the phrenic nerve, has already been described. The most inferior part of scalenus anterior has as a direct anterior relationship to the subclavian vein.

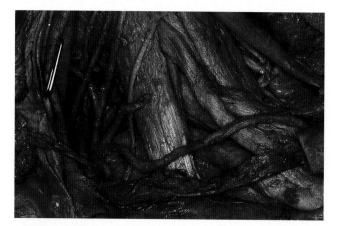

Figure 4-4. Cadaver dissection showing a close-up view of neurovascular and muscular structures at the base of the neck.

Omohyoid

The omohyoid consists of two muscle bellies. The inferior arises from the top of the scapula and passes almost horizontally across the posterior triangle of the neck. The muscle passes posterior to the sternocleidomastoid to join an intermediate tendon. The superior belly passes vertically upward from this tendon at the lateral edge and has an anterior relationship to sternohyoid muscle. The intermediate tendon usually lies over the internal jugular vein and is held in position by a condensation in the deep cervical fascia that ensheaths the tendon and holds it down to the clavicle and first rib. The two strap muscles arising from the manubrium—the sternothyroid and the more superficially placed sternohyoid—run deep to the sternocleidomastoid, covering all of the viscera in the neck anteriorly.

Subclavian Vein

The subclavian vein is the continuation proximally of the axillary vein. It changes name as it crosses the outer border of the first rib and then passes beneath subclavius and the proximal end of the clavicle. The subclavian vein passes anterior to the scalenus anterior and, on the right side, the phrenic nerve. It rests in a shallow groove on the first rib and is in immediate relation to the pleura and suprapleural membrane. At about the medial border of scalenus anterior, it unites with the internal jugular vein to form the brachiocephalic vein.

The brachiocephalic or innominate veins are two large trunks formed by the junction of subclavian and internal jugular veins anteriorly in the root of the neck. These trunks, the left longer than the right, pass downward and meet behind the first right costal cartilage, close to the border of the sternum, to form the superior vena cava.

Thoracic Duct

On the left-hand side of the neck, the thoracic duct enters the confluence of the left internal jugular and left subclavian veins. This lymphatic channel, which begins in the abdomen at the cisterna chyli, ascends through the mediastinum and eventually comes to lie beside the left edge of the esophagus in the superior mediastinum. It lies behind the origin of the left subclavian artery and is in very close contact with the pleura. It ascends through the root of the neck and then arches at the level of the transverse process of C-7, at the peak of its arch rising some 3 to 4 cm above the clavicle. The thoracic duct runs anterior to the vertebral artery, sympathetic trunk, and branches of the thyrocervical trunk. It passes in front of the left phrenic nerve, from which it is separated by the prevertebral fascia, and is a posterior relation of the left common carotid artery, vagus nerve, and internal jugular vein. It sweeps inferiorly from the top of its arch in front of the first part of the left subclavian artery to join the junction of the major veins.

On the right-hand side, a more vestigial equivalent of the thoracic duct entry may be seen in the right lymphatic duct. Lymph from the right arm and right side of the neck are collected and drained into the venous system through this structure.

Other Neural Structures

Two other major neural structures require anatomic description in the area of the base of the neck. The first of these is the vagus nerve. The vagus travels vertically down the neck in the carotid sheath, posteriorly placed between the internal jugular vein and carotid artery. Once the nerve reaches the base of the neck, on the right hand side, it continues its downward course behind the venous structures, crossing in front of the first part of the subclavian artery. From there it enters the thorax and descends through the superior mediastinum, lying behind the right brachiocephalic vein and then to the right side of the trachea. On the left-hand side, the vagus traverses the base of the neck between the left common carotid and left subclavian arteries, behind the left brachiocephalic vein. It descends through the superior mediastinum, crossing the left side of the aortic arch to pass behind the root of the left lung.

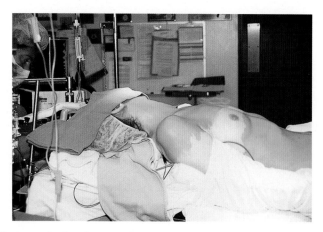

Figure 4-5. Photograph showing a patient positioned in a modified semi-Fowler's position with the neck slightly rotated and hyperextended in preparation for surgery at the base of the neck.

The sympathetic trunk, which has only thoracolumbar efferent nerves, clearly has to traverse the root of the neck in order to supply the three named cervical ganglia. The stellate ganglion, the aggregation of the inferior cervical and upper thoracic ganglion, is located behind the origin of the vertebral artery on the neck of the first rib. The stellate ganglion lies on, or just to the lateral side of, the longus colli muscle, and one of the terminal branches of the costocervical trunk, the superior intercostal artery, passes to its lateral side. The suprapleural membrane separates the ganglion from the posterior aspect of the cervical pleura. Superiorly, several rami ascend from the inferior cervical ganglion to join the middle cervical ganglion.

At the base of the neck, the neck of the first rib and the top of the pleura are almost two vertebral bodies higher than the top of the manubrium. Thus, the dome of the pleura projects through the plane of the base of the neck on both sides. The pleura is relatively thin but is protected and reinforced by an expansion of the fascia of the neck, which is called the suprapleural membrane.

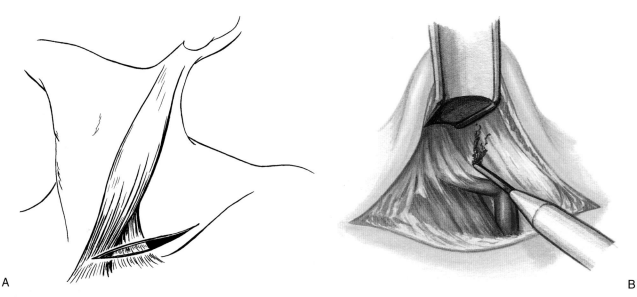

A

B

Figure 4-6. Supraclavicular incision **(A)** and dissection **(B)** of the subplatysma flap.

This membrane, familiarly known as Sibson's fascia, attaches to the inner border of the first rib anteriorly; posteriorly it is attached to the anterior border of the transverse process of C-7. The condensation of the fascia is strengthened by some muscular fibers derived from the scalene muscles. In fact, some have postulated that the anomaly of scalenus minimus may give rise to the spread-out suprapleural membrane as an aponeurosis for this muscle.

EXPOSURE IN THE BASE OF THE NECK

All of the structures in the base of the neck can be exposed through a supraclavicular incision. The extent of the incision, in its anterior and posterior dimension, will be determined by the structures requiring access and whether these lie more medially or laterally. However, if the routes of access are properly developed, an incision that extends from the anterior border of the trapezius to the anterior border of the sternocleidomastoid allows display of the whole of the base of the neck to the extent that the first rib can be removed safely when such an exposure is fully developed.

POSITIONING THE PATIENT

The patient is positioned supine or, on occasions, in the semi-Fowler's position on the operating table (Fig. 4-5). The head is slightly elevated and extended and is rotated away from the side to be operated on. As always, the incision is made with a clean sharp scalpel with the blade held at right angles to the skin. It is placed $1^{1}/_{2}$ to 2 cm above the clavicle, running parallel to that bone. (Laterally, the incision tends to be better placed in a skin crease or one of the lines of Lanz.) This incision is deepened through the platysma to expose the fascial roof of the posterior triangle and the anterior lamella of the deep cervical fascia. The suprascapular nerves are divided (Fig. 4-6).

If it is awkwardly located, the external jugular vein is ligated and divided. Subplatysmal flaps are elevated superiorly and inferiorly as dictated by the exposure required.

The clavicular head of the sternocleidomastoid muscle is divided close to its origin from the clavicle, and the muscle is retracted medially and superiorly (Fig. 4-7). If exposure of the proximal common carotid artery is required, the sternal head of the

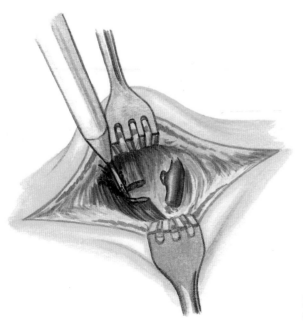

Figure 4-7. Partial division of the clavicular head of the sternocleidomastoid muscle.

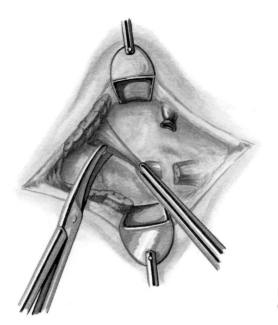

Figure 4-8. Resection of the omohyoid muscle.

muscle is divided. The omohyoid muscle is divided and removed (Fig. 4-8). These divisions are performed with diathermy, using blended cutting and coagulating current. The fascial roof of the posterior triangle is divided in the line of the incision. Skin edge retraction and soft tissue retention are established using a wishbone system of self-retaining retractors. The retention of soft tissue is in three directions—superiorly, inferiorly, and medially—to maximize the visualization.

At this stage of the dissection, the structures on view are the internal jugular and subclavian veins and the scalene fat pad. This latter structure should be dissected free

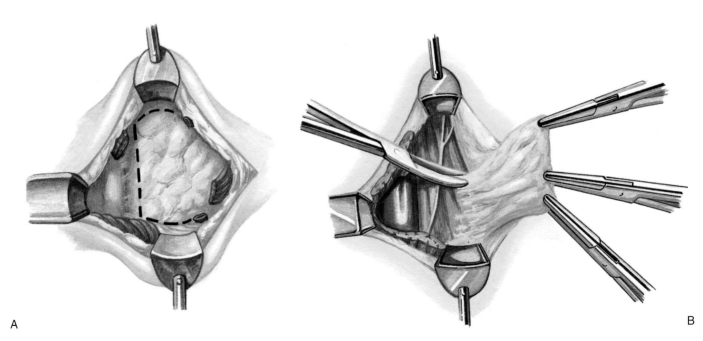

A   B

Figure 4-9. A: Proposed line of incision for mobilization of the scalene fat pad. **B:** Mobilization laterally of the anterior scalene fat pad with the phrenic nerve overlying the anterior scalene muscle.

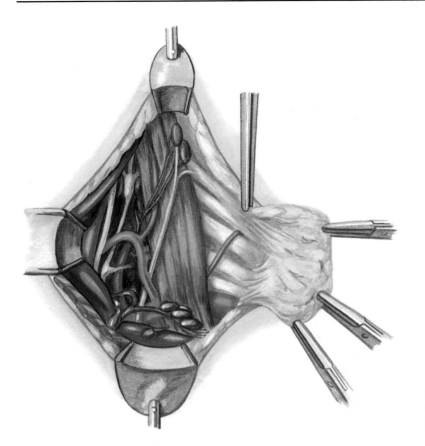

Figure 4-10. Scalene fat pad and jugular vein retracted to expose the arterial, muscular, and neural anatomy at the base of the neck.

of the subclavian vein and internal jugular vein by mobilizing the lateral border of the internal jugular and the superior of the subclavian veins (Fig. 4-9). The fat pad can be retained laterally and superiorly (Fig. 4-10). If the exposure is taking place on the left side of the neck, the thoracic duct is at risk during this phase of the exposure as it enters the confluence of the internal jugular and subclavian veins (Fig. 4-11). This important structure, which becomes a source of a major lymph leak or lymph fistula if it is damaged, must be visualized and preserved. On the right-hand side, a careful

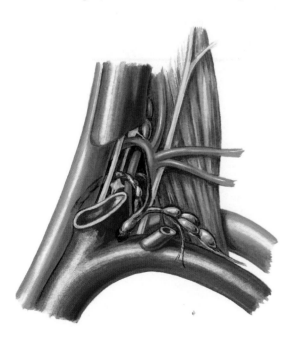

Figure 4-11. Detailed anatomy of the major arterial and venous vessels at the base of the neck and the thoracic duct and its tributaries.

search for the right lymphatic duct is required. The transverse cervical artery and vein are ligated where they cross the field. Any smaller vessels are dealt with at this time.

The lamina of prevertebral fascia over the lower part of scalenus anterior is incised, and the anterior surface of the muscle is cleaned. The phrenic nerve is identified medial to the lower part of the muscle and freed so that it can be retained medially. The scalenus anterior muscle can then be divided close to its insertion into the scalene tubercle. The insertion is always bigger than one thinks, and again, the division is preferentially done with diathermy.

The second part of the subclavian artery is immediately posterior to the scalenus anterior muscle (Fig. 4-10), and once the muscle has been divided, it is easily identified and cleaned of its investing fascial layer. The vessel can be traced and mobilized

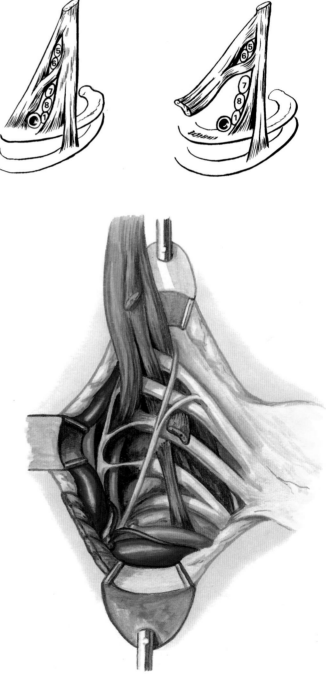

Figure 4-12. The divided interdigitations of the anterior and middle scalene muscle between the sixth and seventh cervical roots (transected muscle). There is also an anomalous scalene minimus muscle originating from the C-7 transverse process and passing in a vertical manner in front of the C-8 and T-1 roots of the brachial plexus.

as far as required medially to its origin on the brachiocephalic trunk and laterally to the first rib. The vertebral artery, arising from the distal end of the first part of the subclavian artery, is identified and traced as far as is required. If necessary, it can be cleaned up to its entry in the vertebral foramen of C-6. In order to mobilize the subclavian artery, the thyrocervical trunk and costocervical trunk can be ligated and divided. Depending on the individual anatomy encountered, the artery can be displaced and retained, either superiorly or inferiorly, as suits the dictates and requirements of the procedures to be performed.

The artery lies on the dome of the pleura, separated from it by the suprapleural membrane. This membrane, Sibson's fascia, is incised. The pleura can be swept downward by use of a folded swab or a peanut swab, allowing access to the thoracic cavity. The pleura may be adherent, and on occasion, the pleural cavity is entered. However, for most mobilizations in the region, the pleural membrane can be retained intact.

Because of the sloping nature of the base of the neck, the neck of the first rib is posterior to the origin of the vertebral artery. Thus, the sympathetic chain can be palpitated, identified visually, and dissected with accuracy and precision through this exposure. Again, because of the sloping nature of the base of the neck, the upper two or three thoracic ganglia are easily removed via this approach.

Thus far, the exposure has dealt with the exposure of the vasculature and the sympathetic trunk. Full exposure of the neural structures requires that we turn our attention to the more lateral and superior parts of the field.

The inferior belly of the omohyoid muscle is resected as it crosses the posterior triangle. The scalenus anterior is elevated and, with the phrenic nerve retracted medially, can be cleaned to its origin on the transverse processes and resected. This exposes the brachial plexus resting on the scalenus medius muscle.

Occasionally, there are small muscle slips from the middle scalene between the roots of the plexus that require division to allow the scalenus anterior muscle to be resected (Fig. 4-12). At this stage of the procedure, the trunks of the brachial plexus occupy the midpart of the operative field. These are then mobilized by careful neurolysis (Fig. 4-13). The previous exposure of the subclavian vessels allows the suprapleural membrane to be visualized throughout its extent, and if it has not already been incised, an incision will allow the pleura to be displaced inferiorly, permitting access to the inner aspect of the first rib. The roots and trunks of the brachial plexus are then fully exposed and can be mobilized further by displacing and separating them from the anterior surface of the middle scalene muscle. When the plexus is free and elevated from the middle scalene, the lateral border of the scalenus medius is dissected

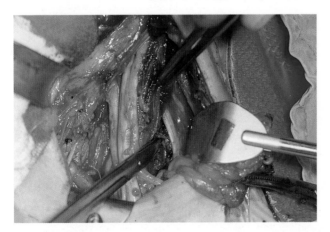

Figure 4-13. Operative photograph of a left-sided exposure showing the major nerves of the brachial plexus, the middle scalene muscle, and the adjacent long thoracic nerve.

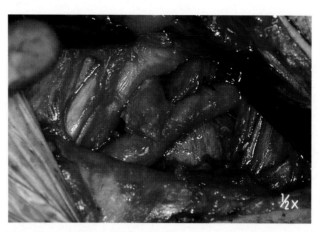

Figure 4-14. Operative exposure of the right neck showing exposure of the subclavian artery and the adjacent trunks of the brachial plexus.

until the nerve to serratus anterior, which exits from the muscle on its lateral side, is identified.

If further exposure is desired, the middle scalene muscle is transected inferior to but parallel to the course of the nerve to serratus anterior, which traverses the substance of that muscle. The mobilized plexus can be retained out of the area of risk, and the long insertion of scalenus medius onto the anterior surface of the first rib, from the tubercle of the rib to the groove for the subclavian artery, can be removed.

Once the scalenus medius is removed, the anterior surface of the first rib is exposed from the neck to the scalene tubercle. This exposure allows safe division of the intercostal muscles and subsequent bony division of the first rib.

Thus, the approach through a supraclavicular incision can be tailored to expose all of the normal structures and anomalies requiring operative intervention in the base of the neck (Fig. 4-14). A precise knowledge of the anatomic arrangements at the base of the neck is necessary, as is a clear understanding of the organs or structures at risk during one of these operative exposures (Fig. 4-15). The major lymph channels and the

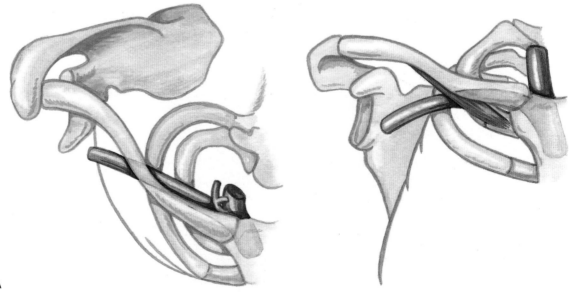

A   B

Figure 4-15. Cephalad and anteroposterior views of the subclavian vein in its course through the costal clavicular space. Note the subclavius muscle in the anteroposterior projection.

neural structures, particularly the phrenic, vagus, and accessory nerves, require a specific search and protection during the exposure.

RESTORATION

When a procedure at the base of the neck involves resection of bone or the large muscles, dead space is created. This is an absolute indication for closed-system suction drainage to be used in conformity with our established principles. In addition, the second obligatory condition for drainage—the potential accumulation of blood, lymph, and extracellular fluid (which is a high probability after large bony and muscular resection)—is addressed by the routine use of a drain in this situation.

The soft tissue of the neck has an abundant blood and nerve supply so that coverage of arterial wounds and grafts is rarely a problem. Viable tissue is readily accessible.

When the brachial plexus is operated on and protection is required in the lateral part of the exposure, the scalene fat pad with its laterally based vascular pedicle provides a ready source of well-vascularized tissue—a "cervical miniomentum." The pad can be split sagittally with satisfactory blood supply in both the anterior and posterior lamellae, used intact to encompass the freed nerves of the plexus, or cover any laterally placed vascular wounds. Thus, drainage and coverage of arterial wounds with viable tissue can be accomplished in the neck in almost all situations.

If the anterior scalene muscle has been divided to provide access to the subclavian artery, simple reattachment of its tendon with two or three absorbable sutures is all that is required to ensure satisfactory healing of that muscle.

Our experience with reoperations on patients with thoracic outlet syndrome has taught us that the scalenus anterior is an "avid reattacher," usually, if there is separation of the cut margins, with substantial fibrosis. Anchoring it into its correct anatomic position not only brings viable muscle over the artery but prevents some of the excessive scarring we have noted when the ends of the muscle are not reapproximated. An alternative approach to this problem is to excise the scalenus anterior. The sternocleidomastoid muscle should be reattached with interrupted sutures along the whole divided origin. Somewhat larger suture material should be used to attach the sternal head to its origin. If there is any doubt about lymphatic leakage, a drain should be inserted between the sternocleidomastoid muscle and scalenus anterior to drain that fluid. Platysma is closed with a continuous suture to align the skin edges, which then can be approximated.

5

Mediastinum

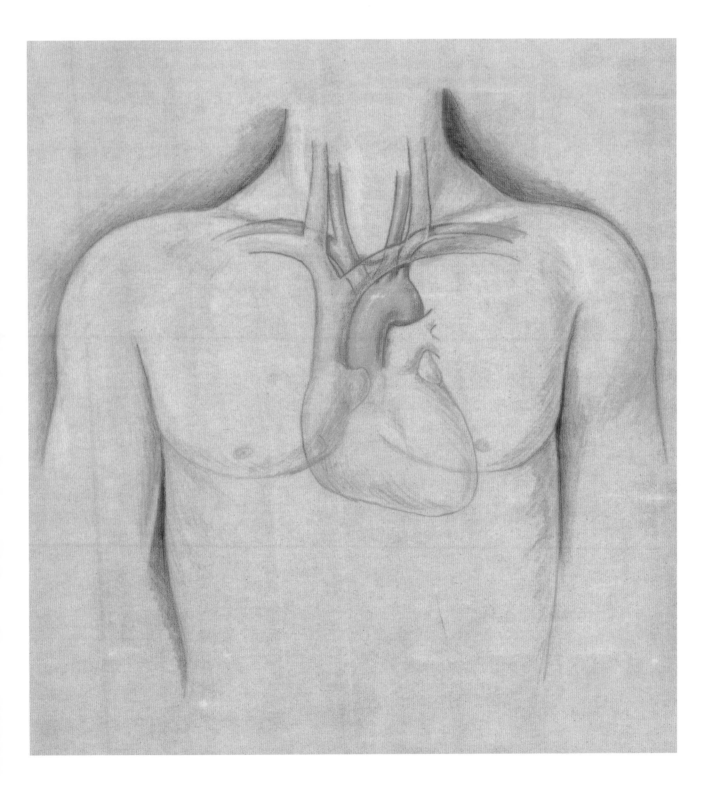

In this chapter we discuss the exposures of the great vessels as they lie in the mediastinum. These vessels and their relations are exposed frequently by cardiac surgeons but only occasionally by vascular and general surgeons. Thus, a review of the anatomy is important before any operative intervention is begun.

SURGICAL ANATOMY

The bony thorax is composed of the 12 thoracic vertebrae posteriorly. Each of these gives attachment to one of the 12 pairs of ribs and their costal cartilages. The ribs provide the bony support posteriorly, laterally, and anterolaterally in the chest wall. The costal cartilages provide the strength anteriorly. The upper seven costal cartilages articulate directly with the various parts of the sternum: 1 and 2 with the manubrium and the manubrial sternal joint, 3 through 6 on the body of the sternum, and 7 usually at the xiphisternal joint. Costal cartilages 8, 9, and 10 articulate with the costal cartilage above, and ribs 11 and 12 have no anterior articulation and are the so-called floating ribs.

The sternum is composed of a manubrium approximately 5 cm in length, a body composed of the fusion of four ossification centers or "sternebrae" about 10 cm long, and a xiphi sternum composed of cartilage of quite variable length.

Some important surgical landmarks are the top of the notch of the manubrium, which is at the level of the T2-3 intervertebral disk. The manubrio-sternal joint at about the top of T-5 and the junction of the xiphi sternum and sternum at the T8-9 intervertebral disk.

The mediastinum is the "central visceral core" of the chest. It contains the heart and the great arterial and venous vessels of the systemic and pulmonary circulation. It also

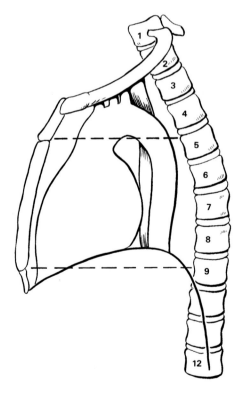

Figure 5-2. Lateral illustration. Bony elements of the thorax are visible with heart and great vessels. *Dotted lines* depict limits that the heart occupies in mediastinum.

contains the trachea and major bronchi and the esophagus. Two major nerves, the vagus and the phrenic nerve, traverse the mediastinum from the neck to the abdomen. For convenience of description, the mediastinum is divided into four subdivisions (Fig. 5-2).

The superior mediastinum refers to the anatomic area above the horizontal plane through the manubriosternal joint and the intervertebral disk T4-5.

The middle mediastinum is occupied by the heart contained within the pericardial sac and is demarcated by the plane described above and a horizontal plane inferiorly through the xiphisternal joint and the T8-9 intervertebral disk.

The anterior mediastinum lies between the pericardium and the sternum. It is occupied in the adult by thymic remnants, fat, and loose areolar tissue, although inferiorly the parietal pericardium is closely applied to the posterior surface of the sternum.

The posterior mediastinum transmits the esophagus and descending thoracic aorta and extends from the level of the T4-5 disk down to the lower border of T-12.

The pericardium consists of a fibrous parietal component and a visceral or serous component, which covers the heart and the roots of the great vessels. Inferiorly the fibrous pericardium is attached to the central tendon of the diaphragm. Anteriorly it is attached to the sternum by short fibrous connections called sternopericardial ligaments and is separated from the rest of the chest wall by the lungs and the pleura. Superiorly the pericardium has prolongations onto the great arterial and venous vessels (Fig. 5-3). In the case of the aorta, the pericardium encloses the ascending aorta to the commencement of the arch, where it blends with the adventitia of the vessel.

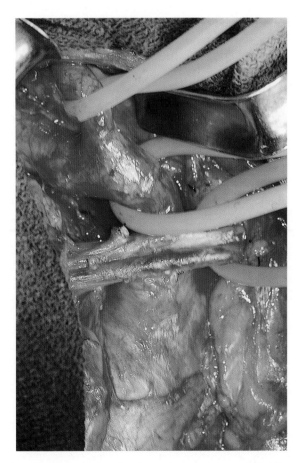

Figure 5-3. Operative photograph showing innominate artery and its bifurcation with overlying innominate vein.

The inferior vena cava is the only vessel to enter the chest inferiorly and has no pericardial covering because of the attachments previously described. Laterally the pericardium is covered by lung and overlying pleura. The phrenic nerve courses caudally on the lateral part of the pericardial sac.

Posteriorly the pericardium rests on the contents of the posterior mediastinum. These contents are the main bronchi, the esophagus, and the descending thoracic aorta. The pericardium is also related to the posterior portions of both lungs and the overlying pleura.

THE AORTA

The aorta begins at the base of the heart from the left ventricular outflow tract. In the chest it is divided into the ascending aorta, arch, and descending thoracic aorta.

The ascending aorta is wholly intrapericardial, and, after arising from the ventricle at the level of the lower border of the third costal cartilage, it passes upward and to the right for a distance of about 5 cm. It has two major branches, the coronary arteries. In its course, the ascending aorta is related to the right ventricular outflow tract anteriorly as well as to the right atrial appendage and the first part of the pulmonary artery. In front of the pericardium at that level is the remnant of the thymus. Posteriorly the ascending aorta is related from below upward to the left atrium, the right pulmonary artery, and the right main bronchus. To the right of the ascending aorta, the superior vena cava and the right atrium lie, and on its left side the left atrium and pulmonary trunk are the immediate relations.

The ascending aorta becomes the arch at about the upper border of the right second costal cartilage near its articulation with the manubriosternal joint (Fig. 5-4). The arch then runs upward, backward, and to the left, crossing in front of the trachea. After it passes the left border of the trachea, the arch is horizontal but courses backward. Finally, the arch turns downward on the left-hand side of the fourth thoracic vertebra and, at the level of the T4-5 intervertebral disk, becomes the descending aorta, which is described in **Chapter 6**.

Thus, the aortic arch is contained entirely within the superior mediastinum. The arch of the aorta is related to the mediastinal pleura anteriorly and on the left, and it is crossed by four nerves, which are, from anterior to posterior, the left phrenic, the sympathetic cardiac nerves, and the left vagal trunk. The latter gives off the left recurrent laryngeal nerve to the left of the ligamentum arteriosum, and the remnant of the ductus arteriosus joins the arch to the left pulmonary artery.

As indicated in the description, the trachea is a posterior and dextral relation. The other relations to the right and behind the arch are the cardiac sympathetic and parasympathetic nerves, the right phrenic nerve, and the left recurrent laryngeal nerve. The esophagus, the thoracic duct, and the thoracic T-4 vertebra are all immediate relations of the posterior aortic arch.

The bifurcation of the pulmonary trunk is found in the concavity of the arch of the aorta just outside the pericardial sleeve; thus, it is an immediate inferior relation. Posterior to the pulmonary artery, the left main bronchus is also directly related to the aorta arch.

The convexity of the arch is the source of its three major branches, the brachiocephalic artery, left common carotid artery, and the left subclavian artery.

The brachiocephalic artery, the first and largest branch of the aortic arch, takes its origin from the upper border of the arch behind the middle of the manubrium (Fig. 5-3). From that origin it runs upward and backward and to the right for a distance of about 4 to 5 cm to a point behind the right sternoclavicular joint, where it divides into the right subclavian and right common carotid arteries. During its course, it lies initially in front of the trachea and then on its right-hand side, where it is related posteriorly to the right pleura. The right vagus nerve is also a posterior relation. The right brachiocephalic vein and the superior vena cava are adjacent to

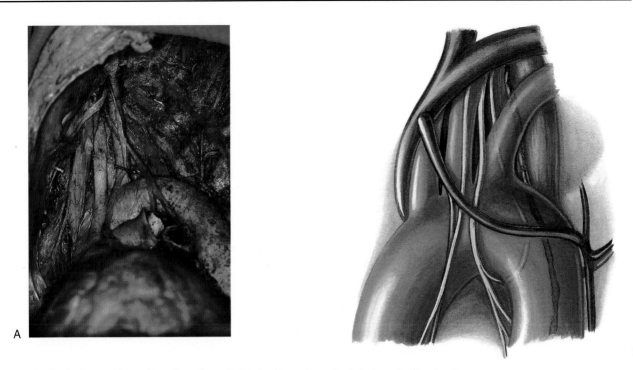

Figure 5-4. A: Cadaver dissection of aortic arch. **B:** Aortic arch and related anatomic structures.

the right side of the brachiocephalic artery, and on the left side the origin of the left common carotid and thymic remnants are related. Anteriorly the left brachiocephalic vein crosses just above the origin of the brachiocephalic artery from the arch of the aorta. This vein is often joined by an inferior thyroid vein in front of the brachiocephalic artery. Thymic remnants in the loose areolar tissue of the superior mediastinum separate the vessels from the deeply placed strap muscles of the neck, the sternohyoid and the sternothyroid muscles, and the manubrium.

The left common carotid artery is the second branch of the arch. It arises from close to the top of the aortic arch in front of and subsequently to the left of the trachea. It passes behind the left sternoclavicular joint to enter the neck, as already described. It has a short thoracic component, related anteriorly to the same structures as the brachiocephalic artery, which it has initially as a right relation. Subsequently the trachea is the immediate right relationship of the left common carotid artery. Posteriorly in sequence from its origin, it is related to the trachea, the left subclavian artery, the esophagus, the left recurrent laryngeal nerve, and the thoracic duct. The left side of this vessel is related to the left vagus nerve as well as the left phrenic nerve and the pleura covering the left lung.

The left subclavian artery is the third major branch of the aortic arch. It arises behind the origin of the left common carotid artery at the level of the T3-4 intervertebral disk. It is placed posteriorly in the superior mediastinum and is difficult to access from an anterior approach. The artery is related to the structures already described in the superior mediastinum, through which it crosses to the root of the neck.

ANOMALIES OF AORTIC ARCH

The clinical description of the aortic arch with three separate and well-defined branches applies in the great majority of patients. However, not infrequently there are variations and anomalies, all of which are explicable on the basis of the embryologic development of the major vessels. Therefore, they should be familiar to vascular and cardiac surgeons operating on this area.

The most common include a conjoint origin of the brachiocephalic and left common carotid artery and the left vertebral artery arising from the arch of the aorta rather than from the left subclavian artery (Fig. 5-5).

The thyroidea ima artery, which is usually a small vessel from the arch, may be present as a large structure and be the dominant supply to the isthmus and lower poles of the thyroid gland as well as the supply to the parathyroid glands.

The two variants of the right subclavian artery arising from the junction of the arch with the descending aorta are shown in the last two panels of Fig. 5-5. This is the site of insertion of the ligamentum arteriosum. The artery may pass behind the arch and be directly related to the arch and the pulmonary arteries or may pass behind the esophagus, forming the so-called vascular ring.

Finally, the arch may have the more primitive (amphibian) conformation shown in panel 3, where there are right and left brachiocephalic arteries.

PULMONARY ARTERIES

The pulmonary trunk takes origin from the right ventricular outflow tract and is contained within the pericardium. It is initially in front and then to the left side of the ascending aorta. It divides at the level of T-5 in the concavity of the aortic arch to become the right and left main pulmonary arteries, which run horizontally toward the hilus of the respective lung.

EXPOSURE OF THE MEDIASTINAL VESSELS

With the exception of the left subclavian artery, the vessels of the superior mediastinum are best exposed through a median sternotomy incision. This routine cardiac surgery approach is simple and safe and can be extended into either side of the neck (most commonly on the right) to allow adequate exposure of the proximal right carotid and right subclavian arteries.

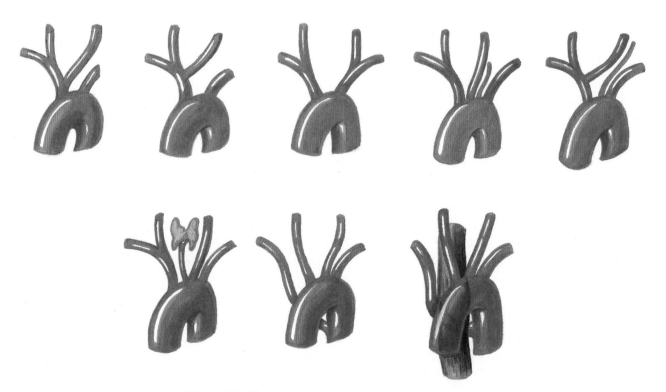

Figure 5-5. Variations and anomalies of the aortic arch branches.

The patient is positioned supine with the head tilted slightly to the left. The skin incision is carried from above the notch of the manubrium into the epigastrium beyond the tip of the xiphi sternum. The incision is deepened at either end to allow access to the posterior surface of the manubrium and xiphi sternum. Then with scissors dissection, the tissues are dissected away from the posterior surfaces of these structures to begin a substernal tunnel. This tunnel is further developed with the index fingers of the surgeon's hands gently displacing the tissues of the superior and anterior mediastinum away from the back of the sternum. Inferiorly, although the pericardium is attached by the so-called sternopericardial ligaments, in most cases, a satisfactory tunnel displacing the pericardium backward can be developed.

Once the tissues have been cleared, a power saw is used to divide the sternum in the midline. It is very important that both the anterior and posterior surfaces of the sternum are well cleared so that the bony division is placed accurately in the middle of the sternum. The saw must not be allowed to wander to one or other side during the bone division. Accurate performance of this division is critical for the subsequent restoration and solid healing of the chest wall. If it is accomplished appropriately, the pericardium and both pleural cavities will be intact in the majority of patients following sternal division (Fig. 5-6).

A critical step following sternotomy is obtaining hemostasis. This is done using a diathermy to seal the obvious bleeding points and to dry the oozing from the periosteum of the sternum itself. Bone wax was once used to control the marrow oozing, but strips of thrombin-soaked gelfoam or gauze have proven adequate hemostatics; these are removed subsequently. The divided bony edges of the sternum are protected with tape swabs. A ratchet-type retractor is used to gently spread the sternum. Judicious use

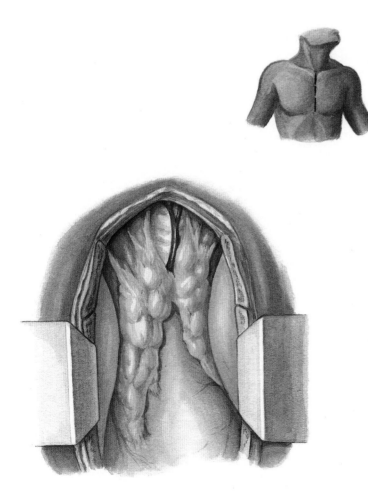

Figure 5-6. Initial exposure of the mediastinum after median sternotomy. **Inset** shows the location of the sternotomy incision.

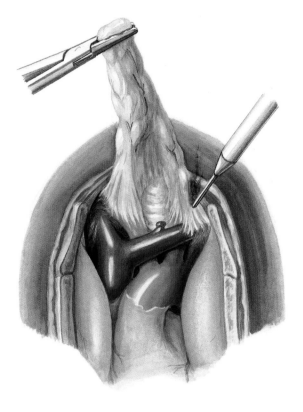

Figure 5-7. Thymic remnant being removed with electrocautery.

of sharp dissection will facilitate the capacity to spread the wound and avoid injury to the pleural and pericardial membranes.

The thymic remnant is elevated and excised, or, in some patients, it may be split longitudinally (Fig. 5-7).

Exposure of the brachiocephalic artery requires a meticulous clearing of the left brachiocephalic vein to allow this structure to be surrounded by a rubber sling to

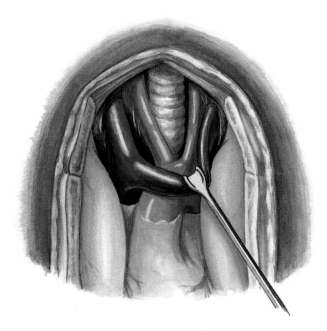

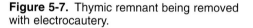

Figure 5-8. Exposure of the vessels provided by caudad retraction of the innominate vein.

enable retraction both caudally and on occasion cephalad (Fig. 5-8). The inferior thyroid vein should be ligated just above its junction into the left brachiocephalic vein. Once the brachiocephalic artery is displayed and circumferentially mobilized, the origin of the common carotid artery is obtained. The appropriate amount of arch is obtained by standard forceps and scissors dissection in the plane of Leriche.

A short extension of the skin incision along the anterior border of the right sterno-cleidomastoid muscle and meticulous dissection upward from the body of the brachiocephalic artery allow mobilization of the proximal right common carotid and the right subclavian artery (Fig. 5-8).

On occasion the ascending aorta is used as a site of origin for a graft. The pericardium can be opened and reflected away from the aorta as it surrounds it (Fig. 5-9).

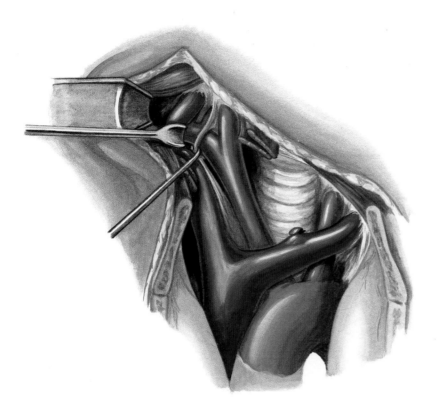

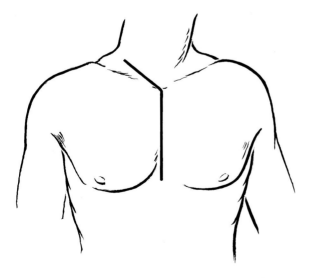

Figure 5-9. Exposure of the innominate bifurcation and right subclavian artery provided by an extension of the incision to the right supraclavicular space.

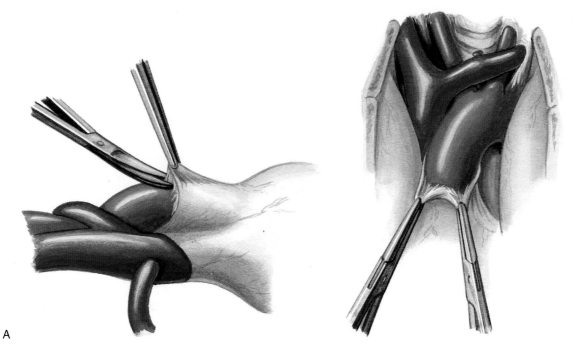

A   B

Figure 5-10. A: Reflection of pericardium caudally in the anterior projection. **B:** Dissection of the pericardium from the ascending aorta in the lateral view.

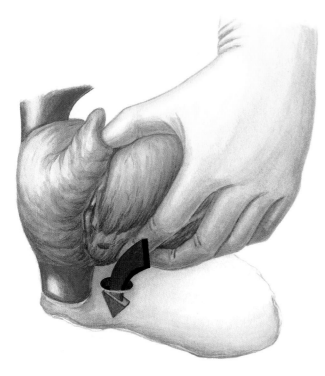

Figure 5-11. Cephalad and left lateral rotation of the heart to expose the base of the pericardium. The *arrow* shows the site for tunneling to reach the retroperitoneum.

This initial incision is best done below the fusion of pericardium into adventitia with the subsequent visualization of the intrapericardial ascending aorta, establishing a clear view so as to obtain the extent of pericardial reflection required for the necessary exposure (Fig. 5-10).

RESTORATION

The key to successful restoration of this sternotomy wound is to ensure an accurate movement-free reduction of the iatrogenic fracture induced by bony division. As pointed out above, the critical issue is the initial bony division, which greatly facilitates the closure if accurately done. The reduction and fixation of the sternal fracture is best achieved by four or five wires passed around the manubrium and the four sternebrae that form the body of the sternum. The wires are passed through the intercostal spaces 2, 3, 4, 5, and 6 immediately adjacent to the bone of the sternum. All of the wires are placed before reduction and tightening.

Median sternotomy leaves a wound with dead space, particularly if the thymic remnants have been excised. Because of the dead space left in the anterior and superior mediastinum, drains are mandatory. Usually two long multihole suction catheter drains are placed to run on either side of the midline from the superior mediastinum and exit on either side of the wound in the epigastrium. Once the drains are in place, the sternal fracture is reduced, and the peristernal wires are tightened to ensure a firm, well united, and movement-free fracture site. The cut edges of the wires are buried so that no painful protrusions are apparent to the patient. The linea alba in the upper epigastrium usually requires one suture to achieve closure, and any extensions of the wounds into the neck are closed in layers. The skin is then approximated according to individual preference (Figs. 5-11 and 5-12).

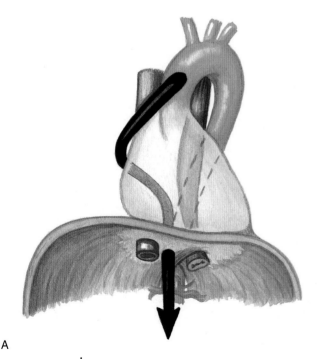
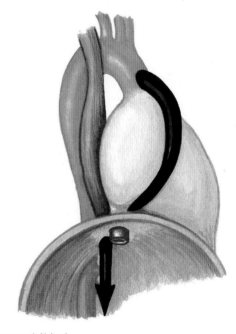

A

B

Figure 5-12. Two views, anteroposterior **(A)** and lateral **(B)**, of the route of a tunnel (*black arrow*) from the mediastinum into the retroperitoneum.

UNUSUAL TUNNELS IN THE MEDIASTINUM

Ascending Aorta to Intraabdominal Aorta Bypass

Ascending aorta exposures through a median sternotomy have been developed in this chapter, and the abdominal aortic components are discussed in detail in **Chapter 7**. The graft is originated from the ascending aorta and is routed over the right atrium and along the right border of the heart but within the pericardium. The exit point into the abdomen is a tunnel created in the pericardium and diaphragm in front of the aortic hiatus, and from there a tunnel can be developed in the retropancreatic plane to reach any part of the abdominal aorta. The combination of the supracoeliac and infrarenal aortic exposures can be used, or if it is required for a multiple vessel revascularization en route, a medial visceral rotation exposes the potential tunnel to its fullest extent.

Descending Aorta to Iliac Artery Tunnel

Occasionally, because of difficulties in access to the infrarenal aorta, the descending thoracic aorta is the site of origin of the graft. Exposures of the thoracic aorta are described in **Chapter 4**, and the visceral rotation components of the exposures in **Chapter 7**. A graft originating from the descending thoracic aorta can be brought through the diaphragm and lie in the plane in front of the kidney to the left side of the native aorta down to the iliacs, where it can be attached to one or other of those vessels. The tunnel is reconstituted by tissue apposition over the graft that has been placed.

6
Thorax

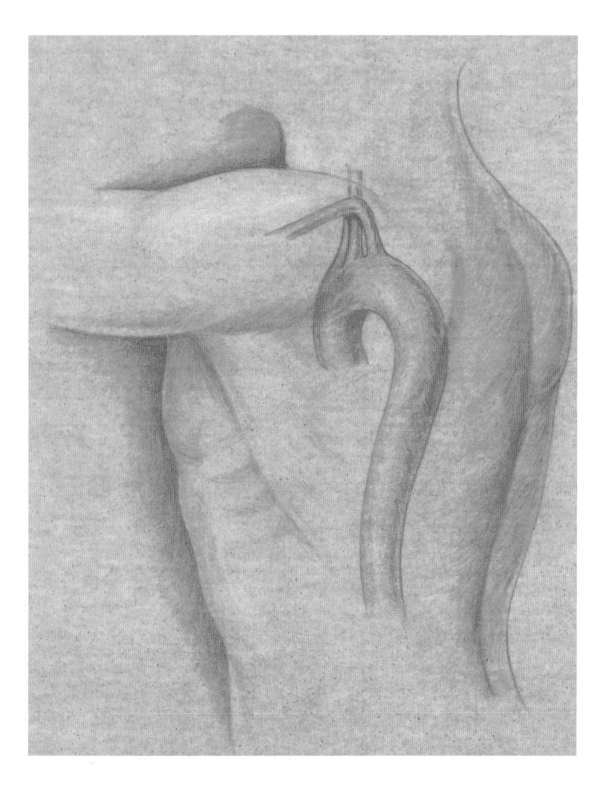

SURGICAL ANATOMY

The thoracic wall is composed of muscles and bones providing protection to the heart and great vessels, the lungs, and the upper abdominal viscera. The bony thorax is composed of the 12 thoracic vertebrae, 12 pairs of ribs and costal cartilages, and the various components of the sternum (Fig. 6-2).

The spaces between the ribs are occupied by the intercostal muscles. These are usually described as three layers: the external, internal, and innermost intercostal muscles. The external intercostal muscles arise from the lower border of each rib except the 12th and are inserted into the upper border of the rib below. The fibers are directed obliquely. Anteriorly, the muscle becomes more aponeurotic and is called the anterior intercostal membrane.

The internal intercostals (11 of them on each side) arise from the costal groove on a rib and insert into the upper border of the rib below. These muscles extend as far as the angle of the rib, where they become the posterior intercostal membrane. The innermost intercostals, which are thought by some to be a part of the internal intercostal, are attached to the inner surfaces of the adjoining ribs. These muscles separate the intercostal nerves and vessels from the pleura.

All three groups are innervated by the appropriate intercostal nerve and are supplied and drained by the intercostal vessels.

The subcostal muscles are small muscular and fascial structures that run from one rib to the inner surface of a rib two or three below. These muscles arise near the angles of the ribs and become better developed lower down in the thorax. These muscles help depress the ribs and are innervated and supplied by the intercostal neurovascular bundles.

The sternocostalis muscles arise from the lower half of the inner surface of the body of the sternum and fan out to attach to the costal cartilages of the second to sixth ribs. The muscle covers the internal mammary artery below the second intercostal space as it passes a centimeter or two lateral to the sternal edge on its path from the subclavian artery to the upper abdominal wall as the superior epigastric artery.

The thoracic cavity is separated from the abdominal cavity by a large fibrotendinous and muscular sheet, the diaphragm. The diaphragm is considered to have three groups of muscular fibers named according to their origins.

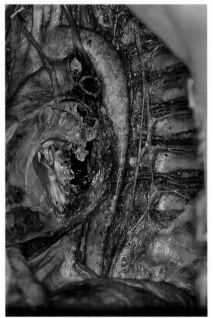

Figure 6-2. Cadaver dissection of the thoracic aorta and related anatomy.

The sternal component is the smallest, being two small fleshy muscles that arise from the back of the xiphoid process and the lower part of the body of the sternum. The muscles enter into the anterior part of the diaphragm.

The lower six ribs on each side provide the origin of most of the anterior and lateral musculature of the diaphragm. The fibers arise from the inner surfaces of the ribs and costal cartilage, and the diaphragmatic origin interdigitates with the origin of the transversus abdominus muscle.

The large lumbar component of the diaphragm is derived from five ligaments and two crura. The lateral arcuate ligaments are fibrous condensations in the fascia over the quadratus lumborum muscles and arch from the 12th ribs laterally to the transverse process of L-1. The medial arcuate ligaments are similar fascial condensations over the upper part of psoas major muscle attached to the transverse process of L-1 and then to the body of the L-1 vertebra. These paired ligaments give rise to posterior and posterolateral muscle.

The unpaired median arcuate ligament is often poorly defined and is a fascial condensation of crural fibers crossing in front of the aorta and forming the anterior boundary of the opening through which the aorta passes from the thorax to the abdomen.

The crura of the diaphragm arise from the upper lumber vertebrae. The right crus arises from the bodies and intervertebral disks of the upper three lumbar vertebra and is larger than the left, which arises from L-1 and L-2; these origins are tendinous, and the medial tendinous margin of both crura contribute to the median arcuate ligament. The crural muscles contribute to the posterior muscle of the diaphragm with the dominant right crus contributing more bulk. Eventually the right crus splits to enclose the esophagus as it enters the abdomen.

From these peripheral origins the muscular fibers extend medially to insert into a strong thin aponeurosis, the central tendon. This muscular aponeurotic structure is domelike in shape, markedly convex upward. The diaphragm is innervated by the phrenic nerve, which supplies motor fibers, and by the lower six intercostal nerves, which supply sensory fibers peripherally.

The diaphragm has three major openings:

1. The aortic hiatus is situated at the level of the T-12 vertebra. This opening behind the median arcuate ligament transmits the aorta and the commencement of the thoracic duct.
2. The esophageal opening in the fleshy fibers of the right crus is situated at the level of T-10 and transmits the esophagus and both vagus nerves.
3. The vena cava opening is in the central tendon of the diaphragm. It is situated at the level of T-8 and transmits the inferior vena cava.

In addition, splanchnic nerves gain access to the abdomen through openings in the crura, and the sympathetic trunk enters the abdomen behind the medial arcuate ligaments on either side.

Above, the diaphragm is related to the pleural and pericardial cavities, and below, from right to left, the diaphragm is related to the right lobe of the liver, right kidney and right adrenal gland, the left lobe of the liver, the fundus of the stomach, and the spleen as well as the left kidney and left adrenal gland.

In addition to these intrinsic muscles of the thorax, some of which must be divided to gain access to the viscera of the thorax, there are a large group of muscles that attach the upper extremity to the trunk that must be dealt with if we wish to gain access to the thoracic cavity. We do not consider here the perivertebral muscles, which are not relevant in obtaining the required surgical access.

The muscles that cover the thorax can be thought of in two groups:

1. Those muscles joining the upper limb to the vertebral column: trapezius, latissimus dorsi, rhomboids, and levator scapulae, of which only latissimus dorsi is relevant to the surgical anatomy of the thorax.

2. Muscles connecting the upper limb with the anterior and lateral chest walls. Of this group the pectoral muscles and serratus anterior are the relevant muscles.

The latissimus dorsi arises from the spines of the lower sixth thoracic vertebra below the trapezius muscle and from the posterior layer of the thoracolumbar fascia, by which it gains attachment to the lumbar and sacral spines as well as to the outer lip of the posterior part of the iliac crest. The muscle fibers pass around the lower chest like a giant fan to converge as a thick rounded muscle, curving around the teres major muscle to lie on the anterior surface of teres major before inserting into the sulcus between the lesser tuberosity and the deltoid tuberosity on the humerus. The lower part of the tendon unites with the tendon of the teres major whereas the remainder of the insertion extends proximally. The latissimus dorsi and teres major form the posterior axillary fold. The muscular fibers of latissimus dorsi must be divided to gain access to the intercostal spaces in all posterolateral thoracotomies. The muscle is supplied by the nerve to latissimus dorsi, which arises from the posterior cord of the brachial plexus and carries nerve fibers from the C-6, C-7, and C-8 roots.

The serratus anterior muscle is a strong sheet of muscle applied around the chest wall between the ribs and scapula. It gains origin from muscular digitations on the outer surfaces of the upper nine ribs. The lower four origins interdigitate with the origins of the first five slips of the external oblique muscle. The fibers of serratus anterior pass backward closely applied to the chest wall to insert into the medial border of the costal surface of the scapula.

This muscle is supplied by the nerve to serratus anterior (long thoracic nerve), which is derived from the C-5, C-6, and C-7 roots of the brachial plexus and descends on the outer surface of the muscle.

The pectoral muscles are the most important anterior connection of the upper limb to the trunk and require an exposition of the relevant anatomy.

Pectoralis minor is a thin triangular muscle that lies on the upper chest wall. It usually arises from the outer surface of the third, fourth, and fifth ribs and the intervening fascia over the intercostal muscles. On occasion, however, the whole muscle may be located one rib cephalad. The origin is near the costochondral junction. It too is fan-shaped and converges to a flat tendon, which inserts onto the coracoid process of the scapula. In its course, the pectoralis minor is in front of the ribs and intercostal muscles, serratus anterior muscle, axillary space, the axillary artery and vein, and the brachial plexus. It is supplied by the pectoral nerves carrying fibers from C-6, C-7, and C-8.

Pectoralis major overlies and covers pectoralis minor. This large muscle arises from an extensive origin. The clavicular head arises from the anterior surface of the medial half of the clavicle. The so-called sternal component arises from the anterior surface of the whole of the sternum and from the costal cartilages of ribs 2 to 6 as well as from the aponeurosis of the external oblique. This muscle is inserted by a flat tendon into the groove that runs from just below the surgical neck of the humerus to just above the deltoid tuberosity. The rounded anterior axillary fold is formed by the lower border of pectoralis major, and the posterior surface forms the anterior wall of the axilla.

Pectoralis major is innervated by the lateral and medial pectoral nerves and is innervated segmentally by fibers from C5-6 and C8-T1. The lateral pectoral nerves (C5-6) arise from the lateral cord, whereas the medial pectoral nerve (C8-T1) arises from the medial cord of the brachial plexus.

Thus, the chest wall is composed of the bony thorax with the intervening muscle and fascia surrounded by large flat muscles that in part attach the upper extremity to the trunk and in part form the origin of the abdominal musculature over the lower chest. To gain access to the viscera of the chest, these various layers must be divided to visualize and subsequently enter through an intercostal space or the space left following resection of a rib.

The major vessel of interest to the vascular surgeon in the chest is the descending thoracic aorta. However, because of its position in the mediastinum, where it takes origin from the arch, which is passing backward horizontally and to the left, the intrathoracic part of the left subclavian artery is best approached directly through a third interspace anterolateral thoracotomy rather than through a median sternotomy.

THORACIC AORTA

The descending thoracic aorta is the caudal continuation of the aortic arch. It commences at the level of the T4-5 intervertebral disk and ends where it passes through the aortic opening in the diaphragm to become the abdominal aorta. The descending thoracic aorta is contained within the posterior mediastinum. The arch, which curves backward and downward, ends to the left of the body of T-4. Thus, the descending aorta has to sweep forward and toward the right to reach the midline by its exit point from the chest at T-12.

The arch contains in its concavity the root of the left lung. Throughout its whole intrathoracic course, the descending aorta is covered on the left side by the left pleura and lung. Posteriorly the descending aorta is related to the vertebral bodies and the hemiazygous venous system. On the right side, the azygous vein and the thoracic duct are related in the upper part of the course, behind the root of the left lung, which is an anterior relation. The root of the lung contains, in order, the pulmonary artery, left main bronchus, and pulmonary vein.

The esophagus has a variable relationship to the descending aorta. Initially it is to the right of the aorta; then, while at the esophageal hiatus at the level of T-10, it is anterior and to the left of the aorta.

The descending thoracic aorta gives off a number of visceral branches, including the bronchial and esophageal arteries. In addition, there are usually nine pairs of posterior intercostal arteries, which arise from the posterior surface of the vessel and run backward to pass behind the sympathetic trunk, which lies over the heads of the ribs. The intercostal arteries cross the intercostal space to come to lie in the costal groove on the inferior border of the appropriate rib. Injury to these vessels is avoided by making incisions into intercostal spaces on the upper border of the required rib.

The lowest pair of posterior vessels from the thoracic aorta are the subcostal arteries, which are distributed within the musculature of the abdominal wall.

The intercostal arteries are important sources of spinal cord blood supply. The dorsal branch of each, which runs backward below the neck of the rib just lateral to the body of the thoracic vertebra, gives off a spinal artery, which enters the vertebral canal through the intervertebral foramen.

Exposure of the Areas of the Thoracic Aorta

Some of the commonly used approaches to the vessels of the chest are shown in Fig. 6-3. The left subclavian artery can be accessed through the neck. However, because of the posterior sweep of the aortic arch, the subclavian artery, the terminal part of the arch, and the very proximal descending aorta are best approached through a left third interspace anterolateral thoracotomy.

The patient is positioned supine and then rotated slightly to the right. The left shoulder is elevated on a small sandbag, and the left arm is drawn up above the head by flexing the elbow and by a combination of flexion and abduction of the shoulder joint. The arm is positioned on a support bar. These movements relax the anterior axillary fold, elevating the inferior border of pectoralis major superiorly. The third and fourth ribs are identified, and a skin incision of adequate length is placed over the third interspace, extending to the posterior axillary fold. Once the superficial fascia has been incised, the inferior border of pectoralis major can usually be cleaned and retracted cephalad, but if required, the muscle can be incised. Pectoralis minor muscle should be divided in the line of the third interspace to achieve adequate exposure of the intercostal muscle. Laterally, serratus anterior is divided along the line of its fibers to

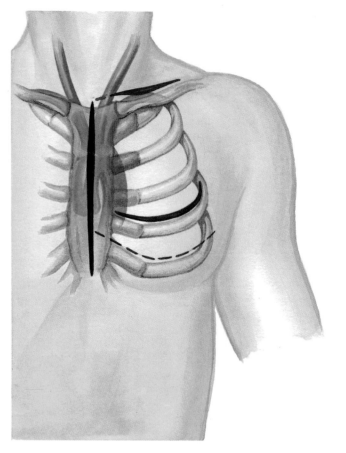

Figure 6-3. Incisions for median sternotomy with extension into the left supraclavicular space. Left third interspace anterolateral thoracotomy (*dotted line* shows left fourth interspace thoracotomy).

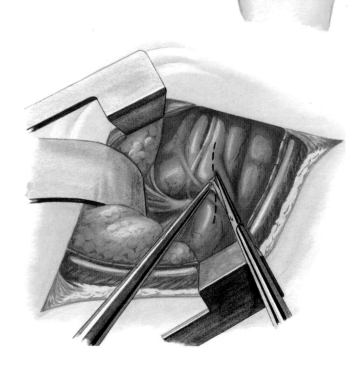

Figure 6-4. Left third innerspace anterolateral thoracotomy for exposure of the left subclavian artery. **Inset** shows position of patient and diagram of thoracotomy incision. Operative detail with retractor. Incision in mediastinal pleura (*dotted line*) exposes the aorta and subclavian artery origin.

expose the intercostal space and fourth rib. The external intercostal is then incised immediately above the fourth rib, and the incision is carried anteriorly into the intercostal membrane and posteriorly as far as is practical. The internal and innermost intercostals are then divided sharply in the same line. The parietal pleura underlying the third interspace is incised and divided along the line of the space.

A self-retaining rib spreader is inserted, and the space is gently opened. The extent of division of the intercostal muscles can then be extended to provide the required access (Fig. 6-4).

The left lung is gently retracted caudally after any pleural adhesions have been lysed. The arch of the aorta will be crossing in the inferior part of the field over the root of the lung. The intrathoracic subclavian artery is visualized passing cephalad toward the left sternoclavicular joint. The arch and subclavian artery are covered with mediastinal pleura, which is incised. Once the pleura has been opened, standard forceps and scissors dissection will allow circumferential mobilization of the subclavian artery and adequate mobilization of the arch.

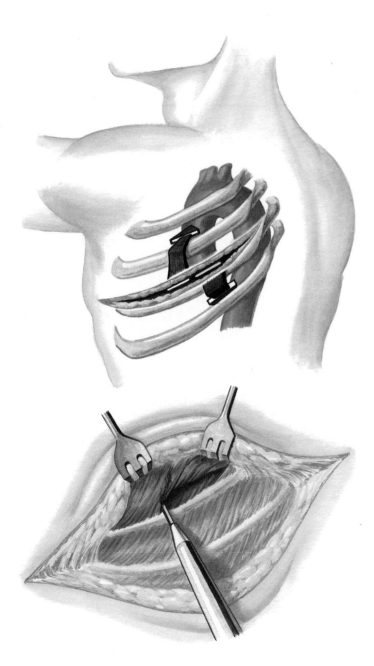

Figure 6-5. Illustration for posterolateral thoracotomy incision at the level of the fifth rib: *upward arrow* shows the course to reach a third interspace thoracotomy; *lower arrow* shows the route for a fifth innerspace thoracotomy. **Lower illustration** shows details of division of intercostal musculature on the rib.

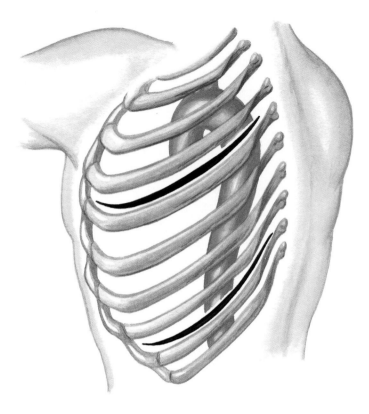

Figure 6-6. Sites of fourth and eighth interspace thoracotomies.

Descending Aorta

Figure 6-5 shows the positioning of a patient in preparation for performing a thoracotomy. Access to the proximal descending aorta is accomplished through a fifth interspace posterolateral thoracotomy, whereas the more distal thoracic aorta is best approached through an eighth interspace posterolateral thoracotomy (Fig. 6-6).

For both of these approaches, the patient is placed in a lateral position with left side elevated. Appropriate body rests are used to ensure that the patient is held comfortably

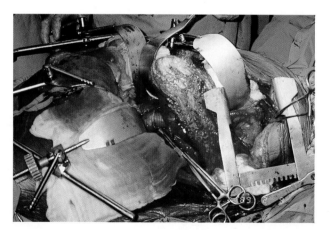

Figure 6-7. Operative photograph of a double thoracotomy at the fourth and eighth intercostal spaces.

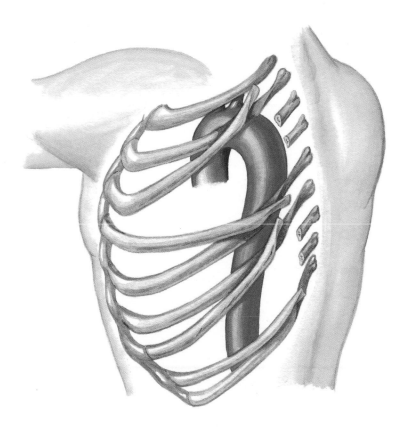

Figure 6-8. Ribs divided and shingled to facilitate exposure after a double thoracotomy.

and securely. If required, the anesthetist may use a double-lumen tube to facilitate further lung deflation, although usually this is not needed.

In both instances, the skin incision follows the line of the appropriate intercostal space. The division of the subcutaneous fat and superficial fascia brings the surgeon to the latissimus dorsi posteriorly, which partly covers the serratus anterior, which is encountered more anteriorly, interdigitating with the external oblique origin. Both latissimus dorsi and serratus anterior should be divided with the diathermy in the line of the wound using blended cutting and coagulating currents. Division of latissimus and serratus provides a clear view of the external intercostal muscles. In these posterior lateral thoracotomies, where secure closure is more critical because of greater movement than in the third anterolateral space, an alternative technique is recommended to enter the space. The periosteum of the rib is scored with a diathermy just below its superior border. The upper surface of the rib is then stripped with a periosteal elevator, and entry to the chest is accomplished by division of the inner layer of periosteum and the parietal pleura. This incision can then be extended for the full length of the rib.

Alternatively, a similar technique to that described above can be used to enter the intercostal space. Usually sufficient spread of the ribs is able to be accomplished, but if required, one or both ribs on either side of the interspace may be divided at its neck to achieve greater visibility after the ribs have been spread by the rib spreader. As shown in Fig. 6-7, the fifth interspace thoracotomy allows access to the upper descending aorta, and the lower half of the descending thoracic aorta is accessible through the eighth interspace. If further access is required, the ribs may be divided at their necks (shingling) as shown in Fig. 6-8.

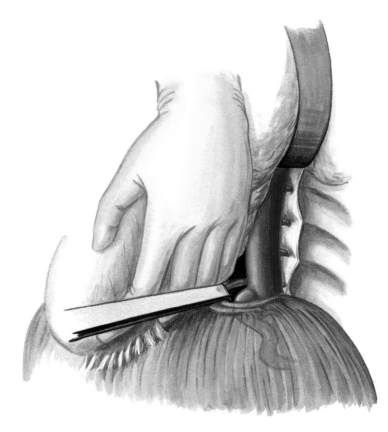

Figure 6-9. Slight retraction of the heart and the mediastinal pleura to complete the exposure of the descending thoracic aorta and the origin of the celiac axis just below the aortic hiatus.

The lung is retracted anteriorly and retained out of the way to allow unfettered access to the posterior mediastinum. The aorta, covered on its left side by the mediastinal pleura, can be accessed and mobilized readily by division of the pleura and careful scissors and forceps dissection (Fig. 6-9).

RESTORATION

Whenever the pleural space is entered, suction drainage to an underwater or similar-type seal is mandatory. Usually if bleeding has been a problem, both apical and basal tube drains are required. However, on most occasions an apical drain is all that is needed. These drains are usually brought out through a separate stab incision in a different intercostal space, and conventionally the apical drain is placed anteriorly while the basal drain exists posteriorly. These drains remove both air and blood and serous fluid.

For reconstituting the chest wall, there is an advantage in using the first mentioned technique of entering the chest. The small amount of periosteum and perichondrium stripped with the muscles provides a firm hold for sutures after the drains have been placed. No attempt is made to approximate the ribs closely, but a continuous suture is placed through all layers of the intercostal space that has been entered, and the suture is passed through the external intercostal muscle or membrane of the space below. If a synthetic absorbable suture is used once the whole length of the wound has been loosely sewn, the ribs may be approximated and the sutures drawn up and tied to act as a long imbrication.

This technique provides firm closure of the intercostal muscle. Other techniques have involved not sewing the intercostal muscle and using perichondral or pericostal sutures to hold the ribs in approximation. In an engineering sense, these techniques are less appealing than the imbrication described immediately above. No attempt is made to reconstitute the pleura, which, like all serous membranes, rapidly regenerates. When the intercostal space has been reconstituted, serratus anterior and latissimus dorsi muscles are reconstituted using the appropriate sized absorbable suture material. The subcutaneous layer is approximated with continuous absorbable suture, and the skin is closed.

7
Abdomen

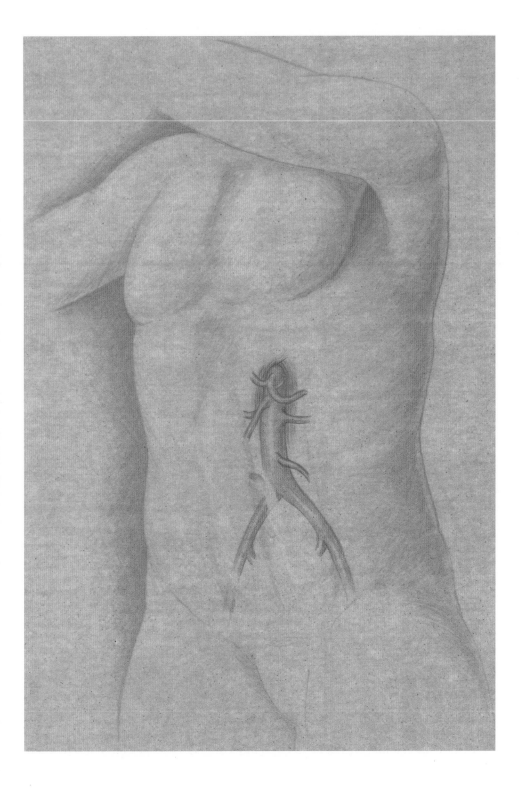

The abdomen contains much of the viscera in humans. These viscera are protected by the lower thoracic cage superiorly, the lumbar vertebral column posteriorly and the large bones of the sacrum and pelvis inferiorly. Joining these bones are a series of strong, highly specialized muscle groups that must protect the organs and initiate the movements of the trunk while allowing it to be flexible and supple. The abdominal cavity is capped by the large domelike fibromuscular diaphragm and is supported in the pelvis by another strong muscular diaphragm—the pelvic diaphragm—made up of the levator ani and coccygeus muscles.

The lumbar vertebrae are the largest of the spinal vertebrae. They have big vertebral bodies with strong intervertebral disks. The transverse processes are large and flat, whereas the spinous process is strong and keellike in structure. The spinous process is surrounded on either side by the erector spinae group of muscles throughout the whole of the lumbar region. A strong fascia covers the erector spinae and joins with another band of fibrous tissue from the lumbar transverse processes and the fascia over the quadratus lumborum to form the thoracolumbar fascia. The fascia extends from the lateral arcuate ligament to the iliolumbar ligaments. Its posterior lamella extends from the iliac crest to the 12th rib.

THE ABDOMINAL MUSCLES

The abdominal muscles are described as posterior and anterolateral groups. Posteriorly the muscles are quadratus lumborum, psoas major and minor, and iliacus.

Quadratus Lumborum

Quadratus lumborum is, as its name implies, roughly quadrilateral in shape. It arises from the iliolumbar ligament and iliac crest and proceeds cephalad to insert into the lower border of rib 12 and to the apex of the transverse process of the upper four lumbar vertebrae. It is innervated segmentally by T-12 and L-1 to L-4.

Psoas Major

Psoas major arises from the anterior surface and lower border of the transverse processes of L-1 to L-5. It also arises from the bodies of T-12 to L-5, the intervening intervertebral disks, and from a series of tendinous arches that extend from the upper to the lower border of each individual lumbar vertebra. The muscle, which is long and fusiform in shape, coalesces into a tendon that inserts into the lesser trochanter of the femur.

Iliacus

Iliacus is a triangular muscle in the iliac fossa. It arises from the upper two-thirds of iliac fossa, the inner lip of the iliac crest, from the sacroiliac ligaments, and from the sacrum. Its fibers coalesce to join the psoas tendon and further attach to the femur. These three major muscles form the posterior muscles of the abdominal and pelvic cavities.

Rectus Abdominis

Anteriorly the abdominal wall has a thick strong muscle, the rectus abdominis. Surrounded by aponeuroses of the lateral abdominal wall muscles, this muscle arises from the pubic crest and the symphysis pubis. It ascends to be inserted into the anterior surfaces of the costal cartilages of ribs 5, 6, and 7 in a horizontal line. The muscle has three tendinous insertions above the umbilicus. The lateral musculature is "laminated" for lightness, flexibility, and strength. It consists of three layers of muscle.

External Oblique Muscle

The external oblique is the most superficial of the anterolateral muscles. It arises by muscular digitations from the outer surface of the lower six ribs, where it interdigitates with the origin of serratus anterior and latissimus dorsi. From the origin the fibers pass downward and toward the midline. The posterior fibers anterior to the free posterior edge gain attachment to the outer border of the iliac crest as muscle fibers. No muscle fibers pass below the line joining the anterior superior iliac spine to the umbilicus, and the muscle fibers tend to stop at the junction of the lateral and anterior aspects of the abdominal wall. The muscle fibers gain insertion into a strong thin aponeurosis that covers the whole of the front of the abdomen, lying always in front of the rectus abdominis. In the midline, the external oblique aponeurotic fibers cross and intermingle with fibers of the opposite side to form a raphe called the linea alba, which extends from the xiphisternum above to the pubis below.

The lower part of the aponeurosis is thickened and folded back on itself to become the inguinal ligament, which extends from the anterior superior iliac spine to the pubic tubercle. At its medial attachment, a part of the aponeurosis is reflected to the pubis to become the lacunar ligament.

The external oblique muscle is innervated by the lowest six thoracic nerves.

A discussion of the inguinal canal and its embryology and formation is clearly beyond the scope of this text. Thus, the relationships of the inguinal canal are not considered further.

Internal Oblique Muscle

The internal oblique is the middle of the three muscles. It arises from the thoracolumbar fascia, the anterior two-thirds of the iliac crest, and the lateral two-thirds of the inguinal ligament. This origin is muscular. The posterior fibers pass generally upward to be inserted into the lowest four ribs as muscle. The middle fibers diverge to become an aponeurosis just lateral to the rectus abdominis muscle. In the upper two-thirds of the abdomen, this aponeurosis splits into two components or lamellae that surround the rectus abdominis before once again joining in the midline in the linea alba. In the lowest one-third of the abdomen, the aponeurotic fibers of the internal oblique all pass anterior to the rectus muscle. In the lower chest the aponeurosis is attached to the costal cartilages of ribs 7, 8, and 9.

The lowest group of fibers of the internal oblique, those arising from the inguinal ligament, arch medially and downward across the structures of the spermatic cord or round ligament of the uterus and give off some muscular slips, which form the cremaster muscle. The fibers then become aponeurotic and arch toward the pubis, where they become conjoined with the aponeurosis of transversus abdominis to insert into the pubis as the conjoint tendon. The muscle is innervated segmentally by the lowest six thoracic nerves and L-1.

Transversus Abdominis

The transversus abdominis is the innermost of the three anterolateral muscles. It arises from the thoracolumbar fascia, the anterior two-thirds of the inner border of the iliac crest, and the lateral one-third of the inguinal ligament. The origin of the muscle is muscular. The transversus also takes a muscular origin from the inner surface of the lowest six ribs and costal cartilages, interdigitating there with the costal origins of the diaphragm. The fibers of the muscle run horizontally to become aponeurotic at a variable distance from the rectus sheath. For the upper three-quarters of the midline, the aponeurosis of transversus abdominis passes behind the rectus abdominis. For the lowest one-quarter, approximately half-way between the umbilicus and the pubis, it passes in front of the rectus muscle. Thus, the posterior rectus sheath has no aponeurotic component below the linea semilunaris formed by that transition. This muscle is also innervated segmentally by the lowest six thoracic and first lumbar nerves.

Following the general anatomic principle of fusion of similar structures when they come together, the various aponeuroses fuse to form the elements of the rectus sheath. The anterior rectus sheath also fuses to the tendinous intersections of that muscle. The posterior rectus sheath has no connection to the rectus muscle and transmits the continuation of the internal mammary thoracic artery, the superior epigastric artery, and the inferior epigastric artery, which anastomose within the confines of the posterior sheath.

The whole of the abdominal cavity is lined by a connective tissue layer called the fascia transversalis, which is more prominent is some parts than others. The parietal peritoneum is immediately subjacent to this fascia.

THE ABDOMINAL AND PELVIC ARTERIAL TREE

The abdominal aorta begins in the midline, where it transverses the aortic opening in the diaphragm at the level of T-12 (Fig. 7-2). The aorta bifurcates to form the two common iliac arteries on the body of L-4, usually slightly to the left of the midline.

Immediately to the right of the aorta, the vena cava accompanies the aorta for much of its course (Fig. 7-3). The inferior vena cava begins by the joining of the two common iliac veins on the body of the L-5 vertebra. It passes cephalad to the right side of the aorta in front of the vertebral column and in the upper abdomen in front of the right psoas muscle and sympathetic chain. Higher still, the cava is related to the right crus of the diaphragm and passes through a groove on the posterior surface of the liver to reach the central tendon of the diaphragm, piercing it at the level of the T-8 vertebra.

Thus, the two great vessels of the systematic circulation are closely related on the front of the vertebral bodies for much of their intraabdominal course. They also share a number of common relationships (Fig. 7-4).

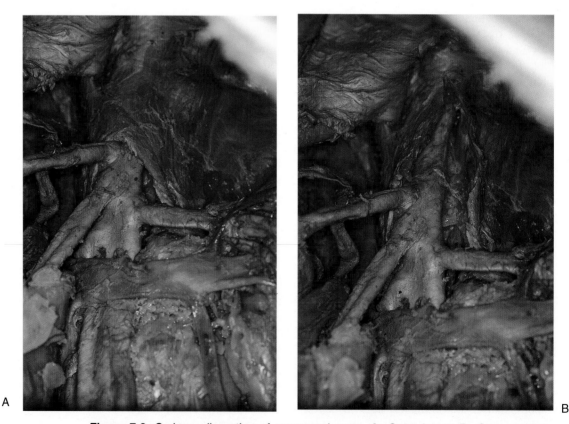

A   B

Figure 7-2. Cadaver dissection of suprarenal aorta. **A:** Crura intact. **B:** Crura open to expose the distal thoracic aorta.

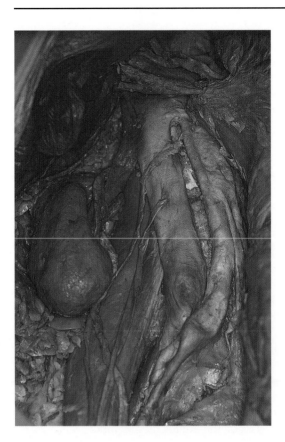

Figure 7-3. Cadaver dissection of right medial visceral rotation showing right kidney and retroperitineum.

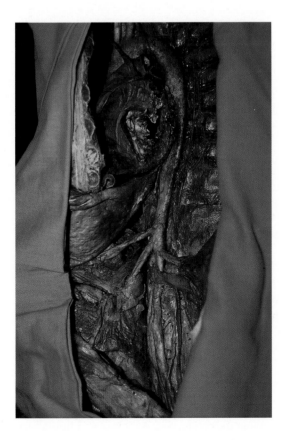

Figure 7-4. Cadaver dissection showing left medial visceral rotation combined with thoracic exposure to visualize the entire thoracic and abdominal aorta.

From above down, the aorta is related to the celiac axis and its branches and the lesser sac of the peritoneal cavity. The superior mesenteric artery is the next ventral branch, and immediately below that, the aorta is crossed by the left renal vein on its path to the inferior vena cava. The body of the pancreas crosses in front of the aorta, and the splenic vein is embedded in its posterior surface. These structures lie in front of the superior mesenteric artery and left renal vein. The next structures encountered are the origins of the gonadal vessels. The aorta is then crossed by the third part of the duodenum. Below the duodenum, the aorta is covered by parietal peritoneum and surrounded by autonomic nerves, lymphatics, and some fat. It is crossed obliquely by the root of the small bowel mesentery and its contents.

On its left side, the abdominal aorta is related initially to the left crus of the diaphragm and the fourth part of the duodenum and the duodenojejunal flexure at the level of the L-2 vertebral body.

The additional relationships of the inferior vena cava are worthy of note (Fig. 7-5). At its origin the cava is partly covered by the right common iliac artery. The anterior relations of the next part of the cava are those of the aorta. However, once the cava passes behind the third part of the duodenum, it no longer has peritoneal coverings. Here it is related to the head of the pancreas before passing behind the first part of the duodenum, from which it is separated by the common bile duct and the portal vein. After passing behind the first part of the duodenum, it regains a peritoneal cover until it enters the groove in the liver. In that short segment, the cava forms the posterior wall of the entrance to the lesser sac—the foramen of Winslow.

Posteriorly the cava lies initially on the vertebral bodies and the psoas major muscle, but higher up it lies on the right crus and the right renal, adrenal, and inferior phrenic arteries, which cross behind it to reach the organs they supply.

Branches of the Abdominal Aorta

The upper abdominal aorta distributes about 40% of the cardiac output over a 5-cm segment to the major intraabdominal viscera. This highly protected and deeply placed segment of aorta is the site of much of the hemodynamic action in the vessel (Fig. 7-6).

Once the aorta enters the abdomen, it usually gives off a pair of vessels, the inferior phrenic arteries, which can be an occasional source of irritating bleeding during exposure of the thoracoabdominal segment.

Celiac Axis and Its Branches

The first major branch is the ventral celiac axis, a short, wide vessel only 1 to 1.5 cm long that lies behind the lesser sac. It rapidly divides into three branches.

The largest is the splenic artery, which passes horizontally to the left behind the stomach and along the upper border of the pancreas to supply the spleen. Immediately before entering the splenorenal ligament, it crosses the left adrenal gland and the upper part of the left kidney.

The common hepatic artery is intermediate in size. It passes forward and to the right, crossing in front of the portal vein, giving off the right gastric and gastroduodenal arteries, and then becoming the proper hepatic artery, which passes cephalad in the company of the common bile duct in the free edge of the lesser omentum to supply the liver.

The left gastric artery is the smallest of the three branches and passes upward and to the left to supply the lesser curve of the stomach.

Superior Mesenteric Artery

The superior mesenteric artery, the artery of supply of the midgut, arises from the ventral surface of the aorta about 1 cm below the celiac axis. As it arises, it lies behind the pancreas and the splenic vein. The left renal vein passes between the superior

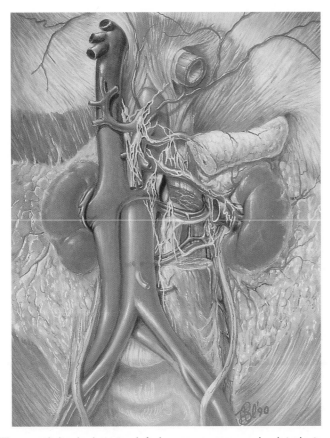

Figure 7-5. Thoracoabdominal aorta, inferior vena cava, and related structures. (From Stoney RJ, Effeney DJ. *Wylie's Atlas of Vascular Surgery: Thoracoabdominal Aorta and Its Branches.* Philadelphia, J.B. Lippincott Company, 1992. Illustration by Ted Bloodhart.)

mesenteric artery and the aorta. The artery emerges from behind the body of the pancreas, passing in front of the uncinate process of the pancreas to the left of the superior mesenteric vein. It crosses in front of the duodenum and enters the peritoneal layers of the mesentery near its root, passing downward and to the right toward the right iliac fossa. It is accompanied throughout its course by the superior mesenteric vein on its right side and, like the celiac axis, is surrounded by a moderately dense neural plexus. It distributes the arteries of supply to the small bowel, cecum, ascending colon, and about half of the transverse colon.

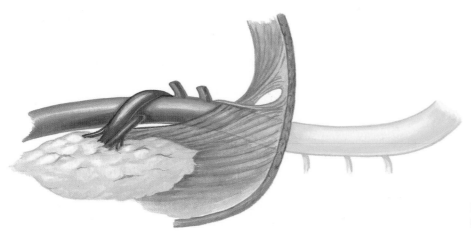

Figure 7-6. Thoracoabdominal aorta and the diaphragmatic relationships.

Inferior Mesenteric Artery

The third visceral artery, the inferior mesenteric, arises from the ventral surface of the aorta about 4 to 5 cm above its bifurcation. It runs inferiorly in front of and then to the left of the aorta, giving off branches in the left colonic mesentery to supply transverse, descending, and sigmoid colon. The continuation of the inferior mesenteric artery crosses the left common iliac artery and enters the pelvis as the superior rectal artery.

The Portal Venous System

The veins of the abdominal components of the digestive tract drain into the portal vein, as do those of the pancreas, spleen, and gallbladder. The portal vein is formed by the coalescence of the superior mesenteric vein and the splenic vein behind the neck of the pancreas and in front of the inferior vena cava at the level of the L-2 body. The vein then angles toward the right, behind the common bile duct and hepatic artery, to lie in the anterior wall of the entrance to the lesser sac, separated from the inferior vena cava by the foramen of Winslow. This vein is usually surrounded by neural fibers and is accompanied by an extensive lymphatic network.

The inferior mesenteric vein, which drains into the splenic vein, is usually seen clearly to the left of the aorta in the base of the colonic mesentery.

Further Aortic Branches

Renal Artery

The renal arteries are usually large single vessels that arise from the side of the aorta immediately below the superior mesenteric artery. They are unusual arteries in that they arise at almost 90° from the parent vessel. The right renal artery is somewhat longer and arises slightly lower than the left. It passes across the right crus of the diaphragm behind the inferior vena cava, the right renal vein, and the head of the pancreas before emerging from behind the second part of the duodenum to supply the right kidney.

The left renal artery crosses the left crus and lies behind the left renal vein, the body of the pancreas, and the splenic vein in a relationship with the left lumbar vein.

It should be noted that the renal arteries and veins supply and drain structures derived from the embryonic urogenital ridge. Kidney, adrenal gland, and the urinary collection system are all derived from this mesodermal origin. These structures are covered anteriorly by structures derived from the primordial "gut tube" contained within the peritoneum. Thus, there is a clear anatomic plane separating the posteriorly placed urogenital ridge structures from the separately derived gastrointestinal tract with its glandular offshoots. This embryonic differentiation forms the anatomic basis for medial visceral rotation on both the right and left sides as well as other variants of the so-called retroperitoneal approaches to the vessels.

Gonadal Vessels

The gonadal arteries are small, slender arteries that arise below the renals and supply the testes or ovaries.

Lumbar Arteries

The lumbar arteries are the abdominal vessels in series with the posterior intercostal arteries of the thorax. Usually, four pairs arise from the back of the aorta opposite the bodies of the L-1 to L-4 vertebrae. These vessels run backward and laterally on the bodies of the vertebrae, deep to the sympathetic trunk, and reach the "spaces" between the transverse processes. They supply the body wall. The dorsal ramus of each lumbar artery gives off a spinal branch analogous to the posterior intercostal arteries.

Aortic Bifurcation and Common Iliac Arteries

The bifurcation of the aorta occurs on the anterior surface of the body of the L-4 vertebra. The bifurcation is to the left of the midline and has a surface marking on the anterior abdominal wall at a point about 1 inch below and to the left of the umbilicus. At its bifurcation, the aorta and the proximal common iliac arteries in particular have an intimate relationship with the termination of the common iliac veins and the commencement of the inferior vena cava, which occurs on the right-hand side of the body of L-5. Because of the direct approximation of the aorta and vena cava, this relationship results in a mingling of the periadventitial tissue. Great care must be exercised in dissection around these vessels, as venous injury does occur, resulting in troublesome bleeding.

The common iliac arteries pass obliquely downward and laterally from the aortic bifurcation to reach the plane of the L5-S1 disk, where they bifurcate into the external and internal iliac arteries.

External Iliac Artery

The external iliac artery, the bigger of the two iliac branches, runs downward and laterally along the medial border of the psoas major muscle to pass behind the inguinal ligament midway between the anterior superior iliac spine and the symphysis pubis. There it enters the femoral triangle as the common femoral artery. Behind the inguinal ligament and lower abdominal wall, it gives off two branches, the inferior epigastric and the deep circumflex iliac artery. The common and external iliac arteries are superficially placed behind the parietal peritoneum of the pelvis and are easily accessible throughout their entire length. On the right-hand side, the only major structure passing in front of the vessels is the right ureter, which crosses the common iliac artery just above its bifurcation.

The proximal part of the right common iliac artery is related posteriorly to the termination of the left common iliac vein, which it crosses, and to the commencement of the inferior vena cava. The right common iliac vein, which initially is a posterolateral relation, passes behind the common iliac artery to adopt a posteromedial relationship to the common and external iliac artery.

On the left side, the proximal common iliac artery is crossed by the major contribution of autonomic nerves to the hypogastric plexus. These structures must be sought and preserved in dissections of that area. The left ureter crosses the bifurcation. On the left-hand side, however, the artery is crossed by the sigmoid mescolon containing the arteries, veins, and lymphatics of the left colon. The superior rectal artery passes in front of the vessel in the base of this mesentery. On the left-hand side, the left common iliac vein is a constant posteromedial relation of the artery.

Internal Iliac Artery

The internal iliac artery is the smaller of the iliac branches. It is an artery of supply rather than a conduit, as is the case of the external iliac. It usually has a relatively short (about 4 cm) main trunk and divides into an anterior and posterior division at the level of the upper border of the greater sciatic foramen. The anterior division continues down in the line of the parent vessel and usually has seven major named branches including the obliterated umbilical artery. The posterior division passes backward toward the foramen, giving off two somatic branches in the pelvis before passing into the buttocks as the superior gluteal artery.

The internal iliac artery has a great capacity for collateral supply, and its branches are widely distributed. Of the vessels that are named, two supply the local lumbar and sacral segments (iliolumbar and lateral sacral arteries), three enter the gluteal region (superior and inferior gluteal and internal pudendal), and one passes to the front of the thigh to supply muscle (the obturator artery). Three of the branches are visceral (the superior and inferior vesical arteries and the internal pudendal artery).

The internal iliac artery is related laterally to the external iliac vein and the wall of the true pelvis. Posteriorly the internal iliac vein, lumbosacral nerve trunk, and sacroiliac joint are its relations. Medially the artery is covered by parietal peritoneum. Anteriorly the vessel is related to the ureter and, in women, to the ovary and the fimbriated end of the tube.

This review of thoracic **(Chapter 6)** and abdominal wall anatomy and reinforcement of the relevant arterial and venous anatomy are important in establishing the bases of the various surgical exposures.

EXPOSURE OF THE THORACOABDOMINAL AORTA

The whole of the abdominal aorta and the lower one-third to half of the descending thoracic aorta can be exposed through a single incision, with the exposure developed according to the principles outlined in **Chapter 1** of this book. This thoracoabdominal incision with a transthoracic and retroperitoneal route to the vessels in front of the kidney makes use of all of the anatomic principles and details described in the preceding chapter and a half (Figs. 7-6 and 7-7).

The positioning of the patient to achieve this exposure is quite critical. Initially the patient is placed supine on the operating table. After endotracheal incubation and the placement of a nasogastric tube, the left hemithorax, shoulder, and arm are elevated off the table and rotated to the right. The shoulder is supported by a sandbag and by soft padding. The arm, which is also padded, is drawn across to the right and fixed in a well-padded support. After antiseptic preparation of the whole of the chest, anterior abdominal wall, and upper thighs, the genitalia are excluded by a sterile towel, and the operative field is draped.

The eighth and ninth ribs are identified. An oblique incision is made from the posterior axillary line in the eighth interspace across the costal margin and the epigastrium to reach the midline just above the level of the umbilicus. If access is required to the distal aorta and iliac arteries, this incision can be carried to the pubis in the linea alba. As in all operations on any segment of the aorta, both groins are available to the operating surgeon in the sterile field.

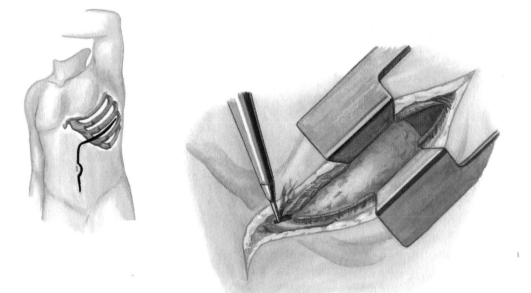

Figure 7-7. Patient position for thoracoabdominal exposure through the midline abdominal incision extending into the left intercostal space. The detailed view shows division of the costochondral junction and limited exposure of the left lung.

The skin incision is deepened through the superficial fascia to expose the musculature of the trunk. From posterior to anterior, the muscles encountered are latissimus dorsi, serratus anterior, and external oblique. These muscles are divided with blended cutting and coagulating current in the line of the skin wound. The fibers of serratus anterior and external oblique, including the aponeurosis, are divided in line with the direction of the muscle and aponeurotic fibers. The abdominal part of the initial incision is continued by division of the internal oblique muscle and the transversus abdominis in the line of the wound. This incision is carried through the anterior rectus sheath, and the rectus abdominis muscle is divided. If necessary, the raphe of the linea alba is divided to allow exposure of the more distal structures. The muscle division exposes transversalis fascia and peritoneum. During the construction of the abdominal component of the incision, care is taken to preserve the parietal peritoneal membrane intact. The thoracic component is completed by a standard eighth interspace thoracotomy as previously described **(Chapter 6)**. The costal margin is divided by division of the costal cartilage of rib 9, usually at about the point of junction of the tenth costal cartilage. The undersurface of the costal margin is cleaned up to the origin of the diaphragm (Fig. 7-8).

Hemostasis is secured in all the wounds at this stage. The initial positioning of the patient allows "a spiral unrolling of the trunk" of the patient, and the skin edges and wound margins are easily retracted by the self-retaining retractor system.

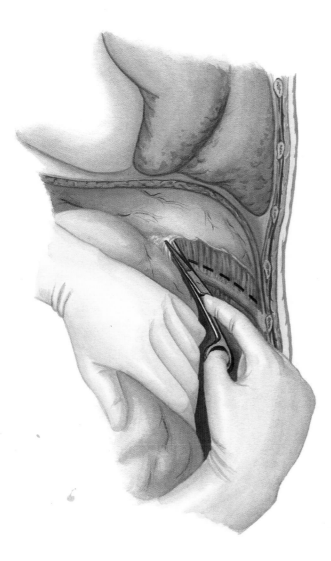

Figure 7-8. The transabdominal left medial visceral rotation is begun. The retraction of the viscera toward the right allows mobilization of the peritoneum off the underside of the diaphragm. The *dotted line* depicts the upper border of the tenth rib.

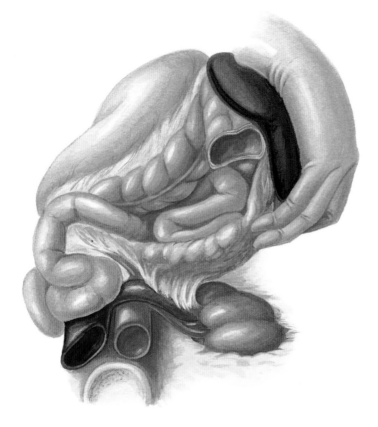

Figure 7-9. Cross-sectional view showing the further mobilization of the viscera from left to right in a plane anterior to the left kidney and posterior to the pancreas.

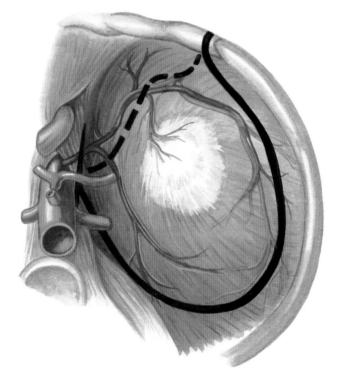

Figure 7-10. Undersurface of the hemidiaphragm showing the preferred pericostal division of the diaphragm sparing the phrenic nerve (*solid line*) or radial division transecting phrenic nerve branches (*dotted line*).

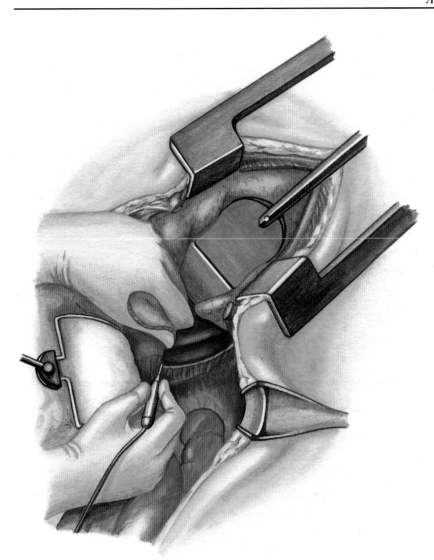

Figure 7-11. Pericostal division of the diaphragm.

The retroperitoneal mobilization of the viscera takes advantage of the anatomic plane of cleavage between the endodermal structures contained within the peritoneal cavity and the mesodermal structures of the urogenital ridge and the body wall. Thus, the retroperitoneal plane is in front of the left kidney and adrenal behind the sac of parietal peritoneum and the pancreas (Fig. 7-9). Establishing this plane is the most important step in this part of the mobilization. Pancreatic injury or postoperative pancreatitis may result if the plane is too anterior, and bleeding from adrenal and other veins occurs if a more posterior plane is entered. The peritoneal sac is gently mobilized away from the undersurface of the diaphragm, and the development of the plane is facilitated by caudal and medial retraction of the viscera contained within the sac. Then the lung is retracted away from the upper surface of the diaphragm. The diaphragm is divided circumferentially from the line of division across the ninth costal cartilage to the spine (Fig. 7-10). The division is undertaken in this manner in order to preserve the phrenic nerve innervation while taking advantage of the dual innervation of the peripheral components of the diaphragm by the respective intercostal nerves (Figs. 7-11 and 7-12). The muscle is divided approximately 2.5 cm from the costal

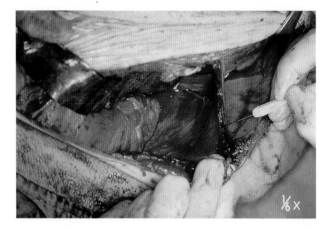

Figure 7-12. Operative photograph showing pericostal division of diaphragm.

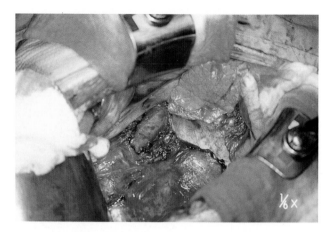

Figure 7-13. Operative photograph showing diaphragm divided but left crus intact.

margin down the lateral wall and across the posterior aspect of the diaphragm until the left crus is reached (Fig. 7-13). The left crus is incised longitudinally in the line of the underlying aorta at the edge of the median arcuate ligament. The incision is extended into the posterior mediastinum from the abdominal component of the crus, from the bodies of vertebrae L-2 and L-1 until the incision line reaches mediastinal pleura along the length of the inferior portion of the thoracic aorta (Fig. 7-14).

The remainder of the retroperitoneal dissection can be undertaken then to expose as much of the length of the aorta as is required for the vascular reconstruction by continuing the dissection in a caudal direction. The medial displacement and rotation of the viscera are completed. The viscera contained within the peritoneal sac are retained using wishbone-mounted self-retaining retractor blades. The left renal vein is cleaned and surrounded by a soft Penrose tube or rubber sling in order to facilitate its retraction, and the retroperitoneal exposure of the infrarenal aorta can be continued as far distally as required (Figs. 7-15 and 7-16).

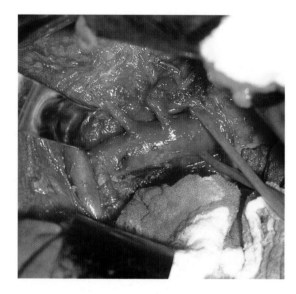

Figure 7-14. Operative photograph showing paravisceral aorta exposed with partial exposure of the distal thoracic aorta.

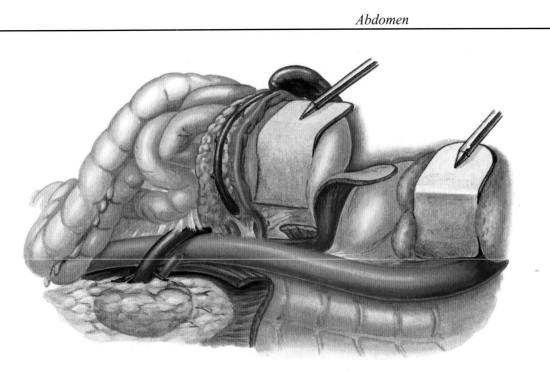

Figure 7-15. Thoracoabdominal exposure employing medial visceral rotation anterior to the left kidney.

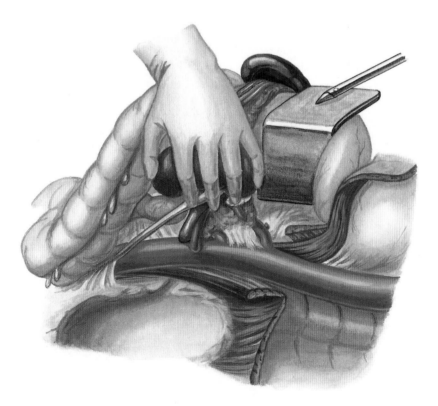

Figure 7-16. Thoracoabdominal exposure employing medial visceral rotation posterior to the left kidney.

Restoration

At the completion of the procedure, meticulous hemostasis is secured. The retraction systems are initially maintained in place while a meticulous repair of the diaphragm is undertaken. This repair utilizes a continuous suture of absorbable material reinforced at 2- to 3-cm intervals by an interrupted stitch of nonabsorbable suture material tied on the abdominal side. When the retraction systems are removed as the repair approaches the site of costal division, the retroperitoneal potential dead space will be obliterated by the parietal peritoneum returning to its anatomic position. Removal of the lung retractor and the shoulder bolster enables the thoracic and abdominal wound to be well approximated, and the completion of the diaphragmic repair can be accomplished without any tension. After appropriate chest drains are inserted, the costal margin should be stabilized with the use of one or two fine wire sutures, and the intercostal muscles reapproximated as described in the previous chapter **(Chapter 6)**. The posterior rectus sheath is reconstituted using nonabsorbable continuous suture, which is continued out to reapproximate the cut edges of the transverse abdominis muscle up to the diaphragmatic interdigitation. The internal oblique muscle is closed, and the external oblique and serratus anterior can be closed as a defined layer with continuous suture. The latissimus dorsi muscle is then reapproximated. The subcuticular layer is approximated if this is required, and the skin is approximated.

TRANSABDOMINAL EXPOSURES OF THE MAJOR BLOOD VESSELS

For most vascular procedures in the abdomen, a transperitoneal approach and route to the vessels is usually chosen. The patient is positioned supine, and the stomach is decompressed with a nasogastric tube after adequate anesthesia has been obtained and monitoring lines are placed.

Access for these procedures can be obtained by a long midline incision in the linea alba with the skin incision extending from the xiphoid to the pubis in most cases (Fig. 7-17). The advantage of this incision is that it is quick to make, easy to restore, and does not transgress any major neurovascular field. The linea alba holds sutures well in its restoration and is a secure low-risk form of entry and restoration of the body wall. However, if the patient has a suitable body habitus with a wide costal margin, a supraumbilical transverse incision allows excellent exposure of the aorta. The trans-

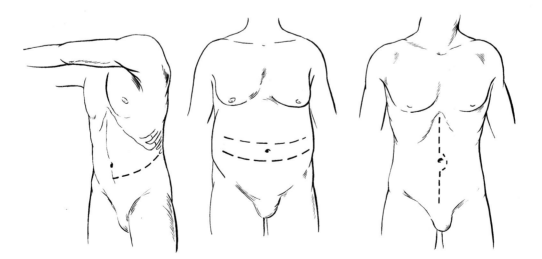

Figure 7-17. Patients in modified oblique (left), modified supine (center), and supine (right) positions. Various incisions are outlined, including oblique flank, transverse supra- or infraumbilical, and full-length midline. All incisions are outlined in *dotted lines.*

verse incision is made in the subcostal plane and extends from the costal cartilage of T-9 on one side to the other. The muscles are divided in the line of the incision. The anterior rectus sheath and rectus muscle are similarly divided. The rectus muscle does not retract within the rectus sheath because of its fixation through its tendinous intersections. The peritoneum is entered to one side of the midline, and the ligamentum teres joining the liver to the umbilicus is divided between clamps and ligated. In both exposures, the wound margins are retracted by appropriately set self-retaining retractor systems. The soft tissue and viscera can be retained as required. As described above, in all operations on any aortic segment, access to the groin is required, and this access is always provided within the sterile field.

If the exposure is of the infrarenal aorta, an infracolic midline approach is usually chosen. The transverse colon is elevated out of the wound and packed off with moist towels. The small intestine is contained in a plastic bowel bag. The small bowel mesentery and intestine and the transverse colon on its mesentery are retained to the right and superiorly using the appropriate blades of the self-retaining retractor. The aorta is seen clearly in the retroperitoneal tissues (Fig. 7-18).

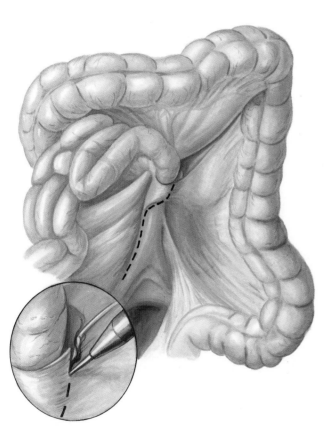

A

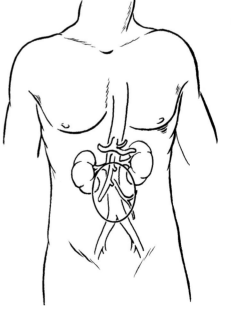

B

Figure 7-18. A: Close up of the posterior peritoneal incision (*dotted line*) being developed with electrocautery. **B:** Overview of the anatomic region of interest. The infrarenal aorta is *circled*.

The retroperitoneal incision is placed initially to the right of the aorta in the groove between the aorta and the inferior vena cava (Fig. 7-19). Inferiorly the incision is extended along the line of the right common iliac artery. The incision is deepened to the periadventitial plane of the aorta, where further dissection and the circumferential mobilization of the aorta occur. The retroperitoneal incision is carried to the left of the duodenum and into the base of the transverse mesocolon. The periarterial tissue is divided, and the left renal vein identified and mobilized (Figs. 7-20 and 7-21). Mobilization of the renal vein with a complete freeing of that structure (Fig. 7-22) is an important step to allow the adequate mobilization of the juxtarenal and, if required, the pararenal aorta. In both occlusive and aneurysmal disease affecting the infrarenal segment, the relatively normal juxtarenal aorta should be mobilized circumferentially. The lumbar arteries are identified and freed so that they can be controlled with appropriately placed bulldog or silver clips. The use of a specially designed renal vein retractor that displaces the left renal vein cephalad allows visualization of the inferior borders of the renal arteries. The right common iliac artery should be mobilized if this is necessary, with particular attention paid to the previously mentioned intimate relationship of the iliac arteries and the iliac veins. The left common iliac artery is mobilized as required (Fig. 7-23).

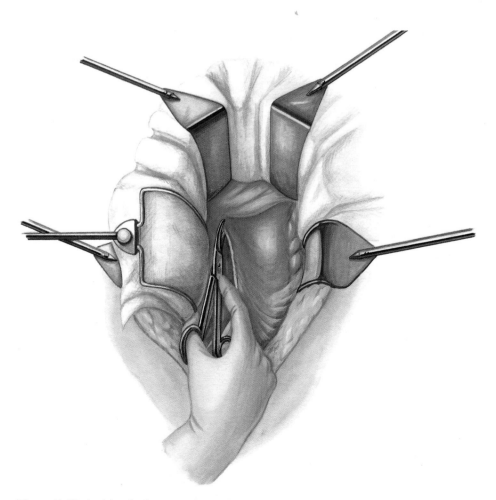

Figure 7-19. Incision in the posterior peritoneum facilitated by the blades of a self-retaining table-mounted retractor system.

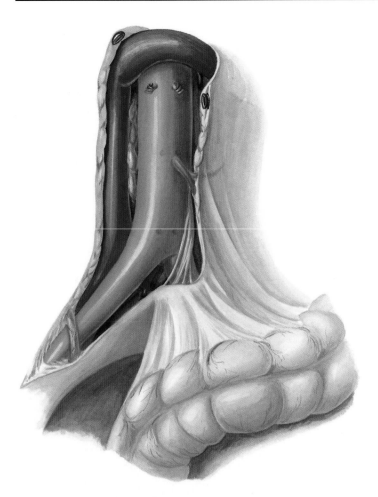

Figure 7-20. Partial mobilization of the infrarenal aorta and iliac branches through a posterior infracolic midline approach.

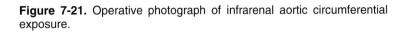

Figure 7-21. Operative photograph of infrarenal aortic circumferential exposure.

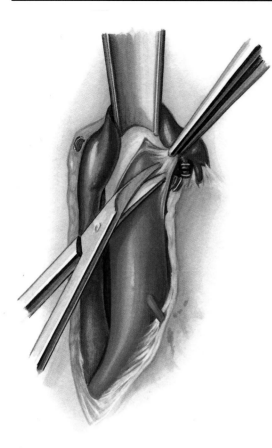

Figure 7-22. Further dissection of the juxtarenal aorta with the left renal vein retracted cephalad.

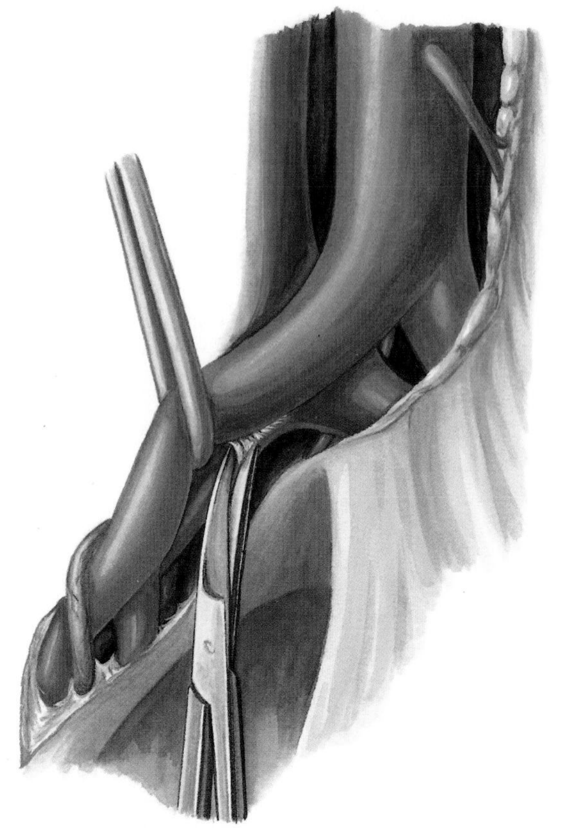

Figure 7-23. Mobilization of posterior right common iliac artery adjacent to right common iliac vein.

If the index procedure is an aortoiliac endarterectomy, the common iliac vessels and the first 2 to 3 cm of the branches (the external and internal iliac artery) are visualized and circumferentially mobilized by extending the retroperitoneal incision and mobilizing the ureter out of the field where it crosses the iliac bifurcation. On the left-hand side, great care is taken to preserve the autonomic nerves that cross the proximal left iliac artery during their descent to the hypogastric plexus.

The left sigmoid colon is elevated by division of the lateral peritoneal reflection in a line parallel to the colon. The external iliac artery is identified below the sigmoid mesocolon and dissected proximally so that the common, internal, and external iliac vessels may be cleaned circumferentially (Fig. 7-24). If the reconstruction is to extend to the femoral artery, standard groin incisions are made over the common femoral artery. The placement and extent of these incisions have already been alluded to; however, it is important to note that the proximal dissection of the common femoral artery in the groin always includes the distal external iliac artery. To this end, the lower fibers of the inguinal ligament are elevated or divided. The circumflex iliac vein is identified, ligated, and divided where it crosses in front of the external iliac artery on its passage from lateral to medial to join the external iliac vein. Failure to undertake this step can cause troublesome bleeding if the vein is injured during the construction of the retroperitoneal tunnel. Mobilization or division of the lower fibers of the inguinal ligament is a very important maneuver to provide access to the deeper structures, and the

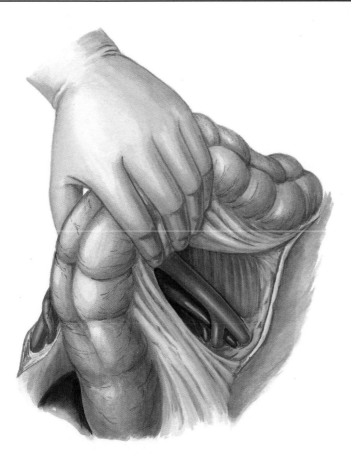

Figure 7-24. Left paracolic exposure of left common iliac artery and bifurcation.

dissection allows the safe beginnings of the abdomen-to-groin tunnel if a graft is to be placed. We believe that division or mobilization of the inguinal ligament also prevents the complication of graft compression where the graft passes behind the inguinal ligament in its passage from the abdominal cavity to the groin.

Retroperitoneal tunnels are best made by the use of the fingers. The index finger of one hand is placed in the retroperitoneal exposure of the right common iliac artery, while the index finger of the other hand is placed beneath the inguinal ligament. The nails of the fingers are maintained on the anterolateral aspect of the common and external iliac arteries, and the fingers are advanced through the soft tissue in that periarterial plane until they meet. Usually one or two areas of resistance are felt during the creation of this tunnel. A very important step is to ensure that the fingers pass behind the ureter to avoid compression of that structure after any graft placement. A long clamp can then be passed over the inferior finger to meet the intraabdominal finger, which guides the clamp into the periaortic wound. On the left-hand side the periaortic component of the tunnel should be made behind the inferior mesenteric artery.

Exposure of the Pararenal Aorta

If required, the proximal extension of the infrarenal aortic component allows safe circumferential mobilization of the pararenal aorta. The important step in this dissec-

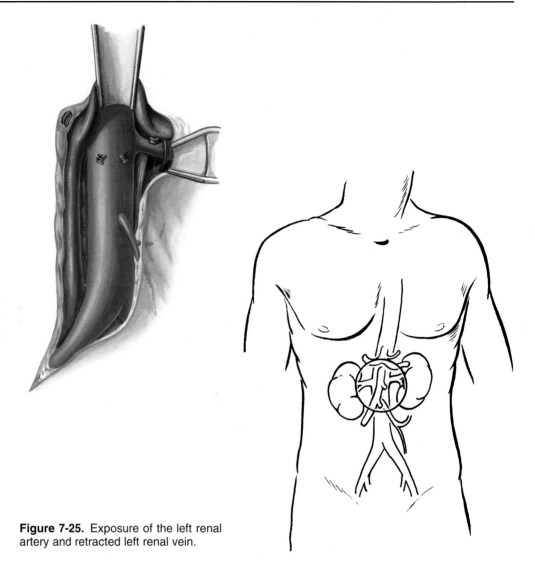

Figure 7-25. Exposure of the left renal artery and retracted left renal vein.

tion is to mobilize the left renal vein completely (Fig. 7-25). In addition, about 2 cm of the inferior vena cava is freed below the entry point of the left renal vein to ensure adequate mobility. When the vein is circumferentially dissected, only rarely is division of the primary tributaries required to increase mobility. The only major structure at risk during mobilization of the left renal vein is the lumbar vein, which is often present immediately inferior to the renal artery. This vein courses forward and joins the left renal vein posteriorly near the entry point of the left gonadal vein. If this vessel is injured, troublesome bleeding occurs.

The renal vein retractor of a self-retaining system can hold the renal vein well cephalad. However, if mobility of this structure is needed during the dissection, a loop of Penrose tubing serves as both a sling and a retractor. The dense neural tissue found on the anterior surface of the aorta is then seen exiting up the field and beyond the inferior border of the superior mesenteric artery (Fig. 7-26). The dissection of this tissue initially requires cephalad retraction of the renal vein, but subsequently caudal retraction is usually required. The origins of the renal arteries can be dissected under direct vision.

The next key step in exposure of the perirenal aorta requires the division of the tendinous components of the crura of the diaphragm cephalad to the renal arteries. The crura are felt by finger palpation on either side of the aorta above the renal arteries as longitudinally running firm cords (Fig. 7-27). Dissection of the tissue immediately

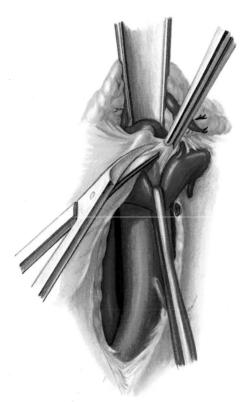

Figure 7-26. Dissection of the pararenal aorta with exposure of the origin of the superior mesenteric artery facilitated by retraction of the pancreas upward.

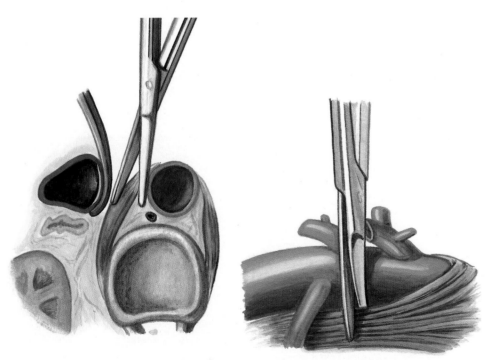

A

B

Figure 7-27. A: Transverse view showing division of the right crus of the diaphragm to mobilize the aorta. **B:** Longitudinal view of the aorta with the left crus being divided.

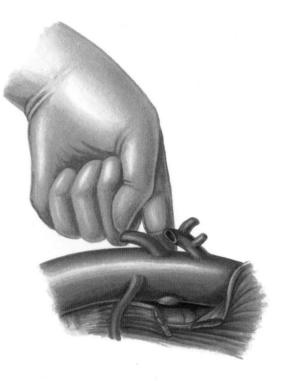

Figure 7-28. Finger mobilization of the aorta after division of the diaphragmatic crura.

above the crus allows the display of part of the crus, which can be identified. The potential space above the renal arteries with the crura intact is very cramped. After division of the musculotendinous structures, however, the space opens for 2 to 3 cm, greatly facilitating finger mobilization of the pararenal aorta and retroaortic space to allow safe clamp placement. It is important to achieve circumferential mobilization of the pararenal segment and to accurately identify the paired lumbar arteries that arise from that segment of the aorta (Figs. 7-28 and 7-29).

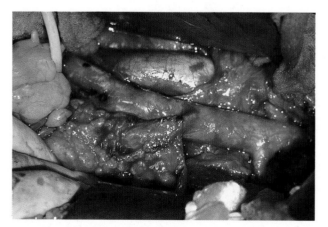

Figure 7-29. Operative photograph showing dissection of the infra- and pararenal aorta and the renal artery branches.

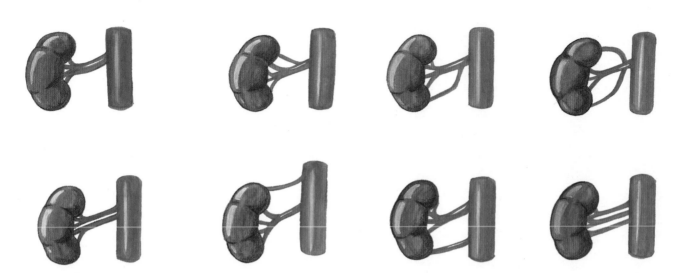

Figure 7-30. Variations and anomalies of the renal arteries.

Restoration

At the completion of the reconstruction, careful hemostasis is achieved in the retroperitoneum. Every attempt is made to use the periarterial tissue to cover the site of graft anastomosis and as much of the aortic wound as is possible. This provides additional viable tissue between graft and/or the arterial wound and the overlying duodenum and also facilitates the peritoneal closure beside the duodenojejunal junction. The peritoneum is then closed over the body of the aorta and along the incision over the right common iliac artery. If the left paracolic gutter has been opened, it is approximated with absorbable suture material. The small intestines are returned to the abdominal cavity while peritoneal fluid is retained in the bag. The transverse colon and greater omentum are returned to the abdomen.

The long midline incision is closed with continuous nonabsorbable suture material, with wide bites taken 1 cm away from the cut edge of the raphe to ensure that the raphe is well approximated without undue tension. If a transverse incision has been used, the transversus abdominis and posterior sheath are sewn with continuous suture. The internal oblique is sutured separately, and the external oblique and anterior rectus sheaths are closed with continuous suture, with the knots of the closure tied away from the midline. In both exposures, it is usually not necessary to use subcutaneous sutures, and the skin should be approximated.

Renal Artery: Variations and Anomalies

Even when the kidney is in the normal anatomic position, the arterial and venous anatomy may not conform to the most common single-artery, single-vein form. Some of the common variations of the renal artery anatomy are shown in Fig. 7-30. During exposure, polar arteries and multiple renal arteries may be damaged, resulting in ischemia or infarction of some renal tissue.

Two important venous anomalies are the retroaortic placement of the left renal vein and the persistence in whole or part of a left caval system. A cause of major venous bleeding during these exposures is injury to the lumbar vein, which often joins the proximal left renal vein. This anatomic arrangement occurs so frequently as to be considered normal (Fig. 7-30).

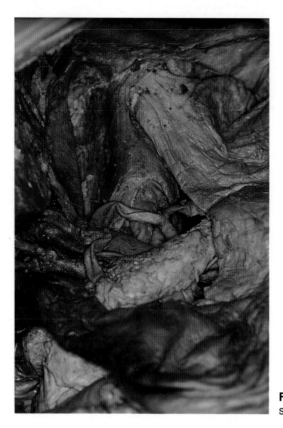

Figure 7-31. Cadaver dissection of the transcrural exposure of the supraceliac aorta.

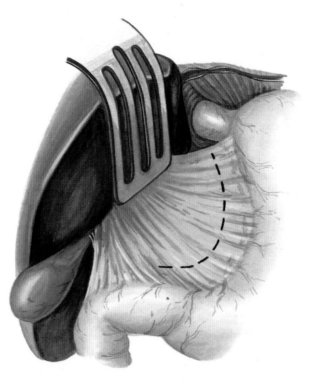

Figure 7-32. Proposed incision in gastrohepatic omentum (*dotted line*).

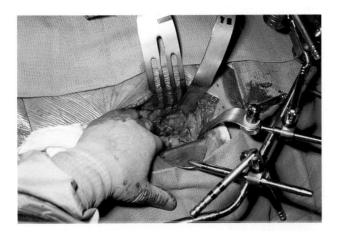

Figure 7-33. Operative photograph showing self-retaining table-mounted retraction system providing retraction and retention during exposure of the supraceliac aorta.

TRANSCRURAL EXPOSURE OF THE LOWER THORACIC AND SUPRACELIAC AORTA

This exposure (Fig. 7-31) and route to the supraceliac aorta can be achieved through a long midline or a transverse epigastric incision. Once the abdomen has been entered, the left lobe of the liver should be mobilized by dividing the left triangular ligament. Once satisfactory mobilization has been achieved, the structure of the left lobe is retracted to the right by being folded down on itself and retained out of the field with a self-retaining retractor blade. The gastrohepatic omentum is then incised and divided (Fig. 7-32). The esophagus and stomach are retracted to the left. The fibers of the diaphragm and the median arcuate ligament are then clearly identified. The diaphragmatic fibers are divided in the midline to expose the distal thoracic aorta (Fig. 7-33). The fibers adjacent to the median arcuate ligament and the ligament itself are then divided to further expose the aorta (Fig. 7-34). This will reveal the dense autonomic nerve plexus around the celiac axis, which should be mobilized and divided. The dissection is carried cephalad to expose as much of the distal descending thoracic aorta as is required for the reconstruction. The dissection then is carried caudally. The pancreas is identified and dissected free of its posterior attachments to allow visualization of the first few centimeters of the superior mesenteric artery. The viscera, including the diaphragm and pancreas, are retained by self-retaining retractor blades (Fig. 7-35). This exposure and route to the vessels allow the complete mobilization of the supraceliac aorta as well as a good length of the descending thoracic aorta in continuity. The main structures at risk during this exposure include the inferior phrenic arteries, which are the first branches of the intraabdominal aorta.

This is an increasingly important exposure for the surgeon to have in his or her armamentarium (Fig. 7-36). In the management of some aneurysms and intraabdominal bleeding, rapid exposure of the supraceliac aorta and placement of the clamp can be life-saving. The exposure should be practiced by all trainees in the autopsy room to become familiar with this rapid, simple, and safe exposure of the distal thoracic aorta.

Anomalies of the Celiac Axis

The celiac axis is classically described as short and having three branches: splenic, gastric, and hepatic arteries. However, because of anomalous embryologic development of the fore- and midgut and the supplying vessels, the celiac and superior mesenteric arteries may share some branches. The common variations are shown in Fig. 7-37.

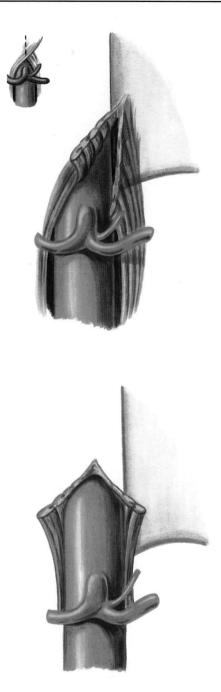

Figure 7-34. Incision of the arcuate ligament and left crus of the diaphragm vertically **(bottom)** and diagonally into the left pleural space **(top)**. This is incorrect. The **inset** shows by the *dotted line* the correct line of the crural division.

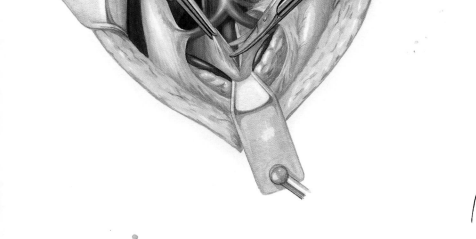

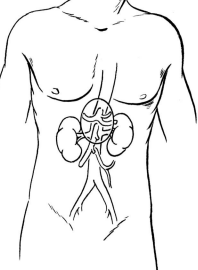

Figure 7-35. Retractor system providing exposure for a complete dissection of the supraceliac subdiaphragmatic aorta.

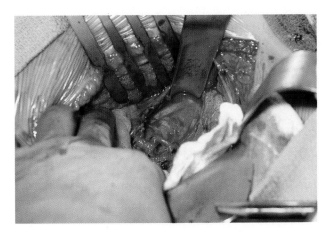

Figure 7-36. Operative exposure showing the supraceliac aorta and branches.

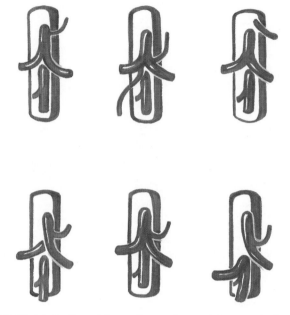

Figure 7-37. Anatomic anomalies of the celiac and superior mesenteric artery origins.

The celiac axis may be a longer artery in some subjects and may arise from the thoracic aorta. In this circumstance, it may be compressed at the level of the median arcuate ligament where it enters the abdomen.

Restoration

After careful hemostasis, the left lobe of the liver is restored to its normal position, and the other retraction is released. Further check of hemostasis is undertaken after the retraction is removed. When the wound is dry, the tissues are allowed to obliterate the dead space. No repair of the gastrohepatic omentum is necessary. Standard restoration of the abdominal wall completes the procedure.

EXPOSURE OF THE ABDOMINAL AORTA AND ITS PRIMARY BRANCHES BY TRANSABDOMINAL MEDIAL VISCERAL ROTATION

The patient is prepared and draped as has already been described. A nasogastric tube is routinely passed to decompress the stomach after endotracheal anesthesia has been established.

The choice of incision depends on the patient's body habitus, with adequate exposure obtained through a full midline incision or a transverse incision in those patients with broad costal margins. Wound retraction is established with a self-retaining system. The small intestine is placed in a bowel bag and retained to the right side.

This transperitoneal approach is converted into a retroperitoneal route to the vessels by incision of the left lateral peritoneal reflection and full mobilization of the descending colon (Fig. 7-38). This line of peritoneal incision is then continued cephalad, and the spleen is mobilized by division of the splenorenal ligament. The posterolateral peritoneal attachments of the spleen to the diaphragm above the kidney are divided. The left colon and spleen are elevated and rotated, and the viscera are mobilized by establishing a plane in front of the left kidney adrenal and urinary collecting system and behind the spleen, pancreas, and colon, as was established during the thoracoabdominal retroperitoneal approach (Fig. 7-39). As indicated previously and reiterated here, this plane takes advantage of the embryologically determined cleavage plane between mesodermally derived and endodermally derived structures. The correct def-

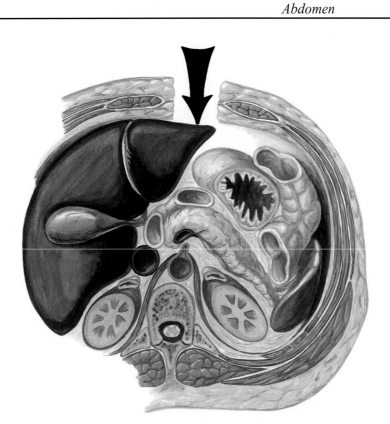

Figure 7-38. Transverse view showing the direction of the midline approach to the aorta (*bold arrow*). Note the overlying viscera at level of the origin of the celiac axis.

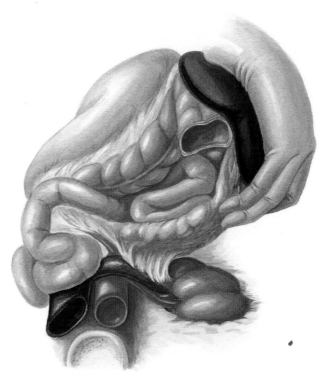

Figure 7-39. Cross-sectional view showing the further mobilization of the viscera from left to right in a plane anterior to the left kidney and posterior to the pancreas.

inition of this embryologically determined plane is the single most important step in this part of the mobilization. As the dissection proceeds, the spleen, the colon, and the tail and body of the pancreas are elevated anteromedially and retracted to the right. At the superior aspect of the dissection, the viscera are tethered by the peritoneal reflections from the undersurface of the diaphragm which must be divided to allow for mobilization of the fundus of the stomach. The viscera are then rotated, allowing complete visualization of the left crus of the diaphragm. The viscera are protected with sponges and retained out of the operative field using splanchnic retractor blades in the self-retaining system.

The upper abdominal aorta is exposed by longitudinal division of the left crus in a fashion similar to that described previously. Following division of the crus, the autonomic nervous tissue is clearly visible and is mobilized and displaced, with resection performed as needed (Fig. 7-40). If proximal access is required, the incision through the crus is carried into the mediastinum to expose the lower thoracic aorta. The celiac and superior mesenteric arteries are mobilized (Fig. 7-41). As required, the distal aorta, inferior mesenteric, and both common iliac arteries are mobilized. Once the dissection is complete and the viscera are retained, the only remaining structure crossing the aorta is the left renal vein (Fig. 7-42). This vessel should be dissected to its junction with the

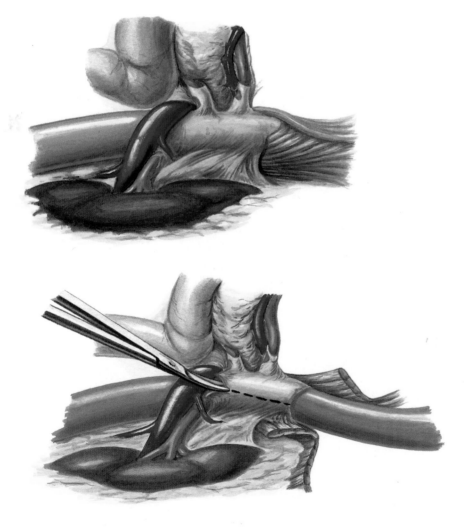

Figure 7-40. Lateral view of the thoracoabdominal aorta partly exposed **(top)**. The crura have been divided, and the autonomic ganglion tissue is being incised (*dotted line*) in the **lower illustration**.

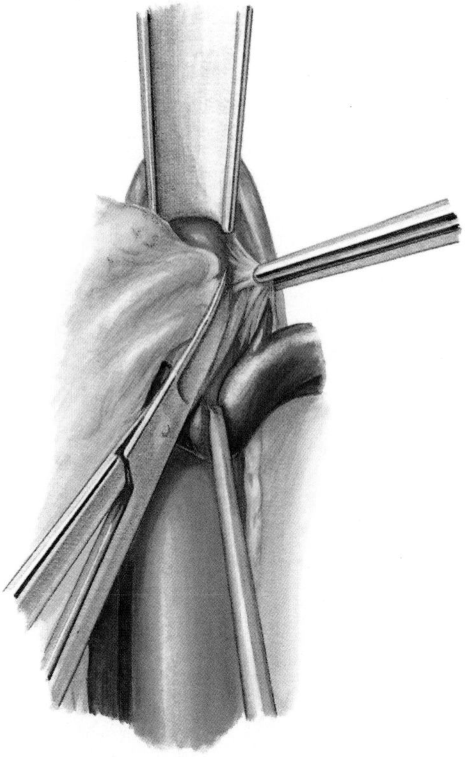

Figure 7-41. Mobilization of the paravisceral aorta adjacent to the origin of the celiac axis and superior mesenteric arteries.

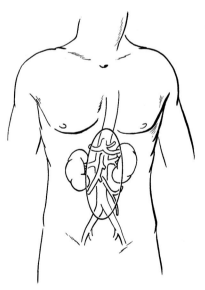

Figure 7-42. Retraction providing exposure for complete display of the upper abdominal aorta and its branches. The entire abdominal aorta and its branches are *circled* in the insert.

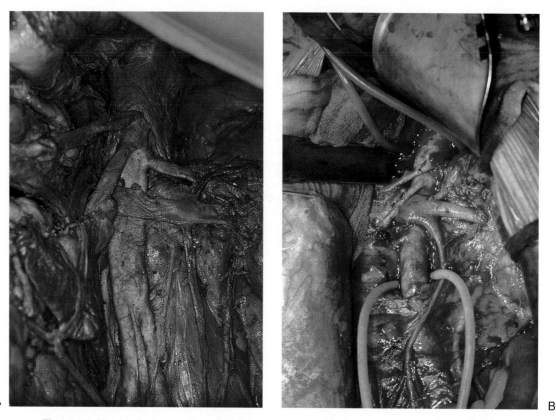

A
B

Figure 7-43. A: Cadaver dissection of the upper abdominal aorta and its branches exposed using medial visceral rotation. **B:** An operative photograph of the upper abdominal aorta and its branches exposed by medial visceral rotation.

inferior vena cava and mobilized so that it can be retracted either upward or downward to facilitate the dissection of the pararenal aorta. The left renal artery is readily seen, and by mobilizing the inferior vena cava and retracting it to the right-hand side, the right renal artery can be exposed for 2 to 3 cm (Figs. 7-43 through 7-45).

We prefer to use the plane in front of the kidney because it has some clear advantages embryologically (Fig. 7-46). Moreover, in patients with aortic occlusive disease, mobilization of the aorta using a plane posterior to the left kidney does not provide good access, as the space behind the renal artery is limited by the spine and is very narrow (Fig. 7-47). In addition, medial reflection of the kidney is incomplete, and access to the anterior part of the renal artery is unsatisfactory (Fig. 7-48). However, in patients with aneurysm or disease of this segment of the aorta, enlargement of the aorta increases the distance from the spine to the renal artery, and the renal vessels assume a much more anterior position (Fig. 7-49). This allows more complete rotation. The size increase and the facilitated rotation present the surgeon with a satisfactory arc of aorta through which inclusion grafting and direct branch reattachment can be performed.

Restoration

The secret to satisfactory restoration of this approach to the vessels is to have chosen and developed the correct prerenal or postrenal plane. Replacing the viscera at the end of the procedure obliterates the dead space and ensures anatomic restoration. The left colonic attachments do not need to be sutured but can be restored with a continuous absorbable suture. Standard closure of the abdominal wall is then carried out.

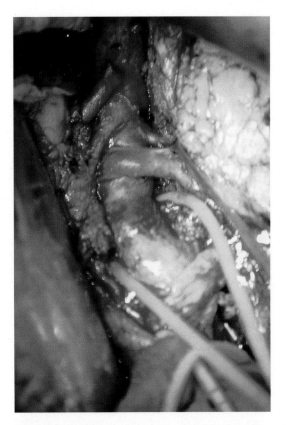

Figure 7-44. Operative photograph of the upper abdominal aorta and left renal artery exposed by medial visceral rotation.

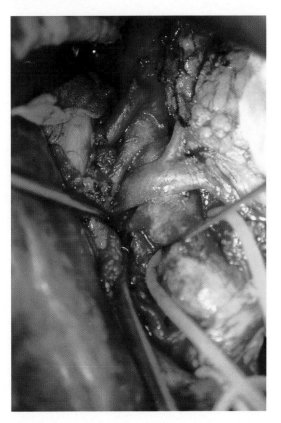

Figure 7-45. Operative photograph of upper abdominal aorta and branches and right renal artery exposed by medial visceral rotation.

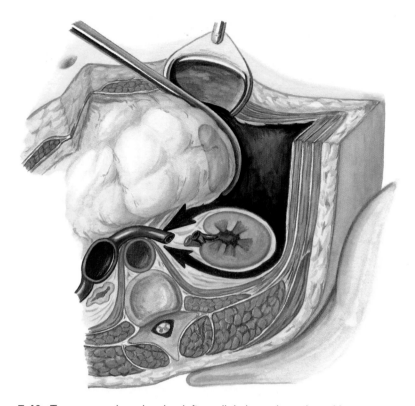

Figure 7-46. Transverse view showing left medial visceral rotation with a route anterior to the kidney (*upper arrow*) and an alternate route posterior to the kidney (*lower arrow*) that can be utilized in exposing the aorta.

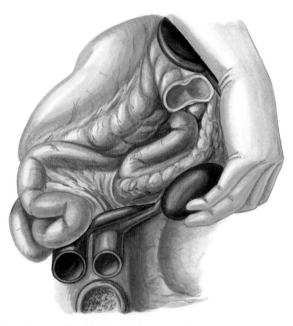

Figure 7-47. Left medial visceral rotation in a plane posterior to the left kidney.

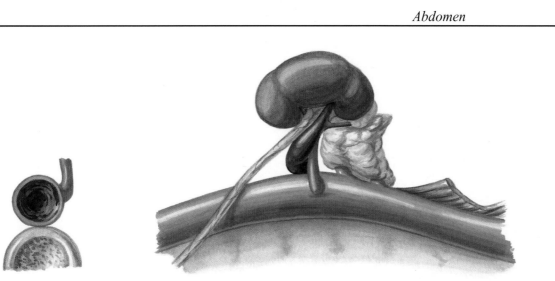

Figure 7-48. A normal-sized aorta being exposed in a plane posterior to the left kidney.

LIMITS OF EXPOSURE

All of the standard exposures of the vessels in the abdomen have limits imposed by the anatomic structures encountered. In general, these limits are terms imposed at the superior aspects of the various exposures.

A long midline abdominal wall incision and a midline retroperitoneal exposure in the infracolic compartment affords total access to the para- and infrarenal aorta and the iliac vessels. However, superiorly the access is limited by the need to retract and work behind the root of and the contents of the transverse mesocolon.

The other approaches described also have exposure limits. These limits include those imposed by the body wall, the diaphragm, and the viscera. The next series of figures explores some of these limits.

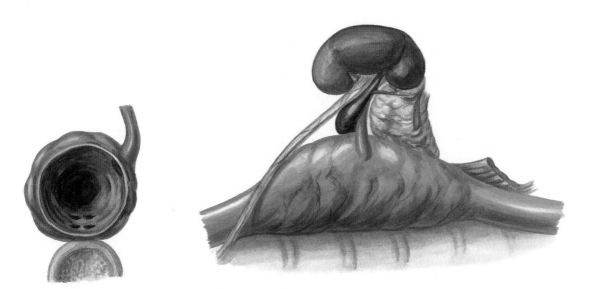

Figure 7-49. Left medial visceral rotation to expose an aneurysmal thoracoabdominal aorta in a plane posterior to the left kidney. Note the ample space between the posterior origin of the left renal artery and the edge of the lumbar spine seen in both lateral and cross-sectional views.

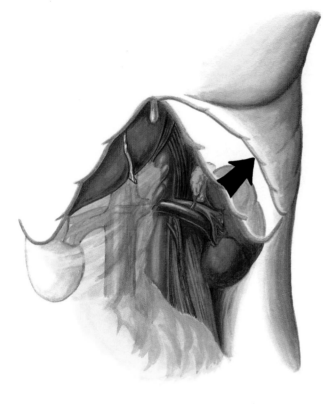

Figure 7-50. Upward and lateral limits of medial visceral rotation through a transabdominal approach. The displacement of the costal margin (*arrow*) is shown.

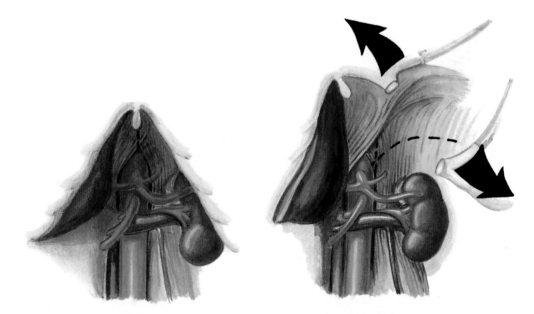

Figure 7-51. Upper extent of the transabdominal medial visceral rotation exposure of the aorta **(left)**. The extension of the exposure into the left chest by left thoracoabdominal incision and by dividing the diaphragm as indicated by the *dotted lines* dramatically extends the exposure proximally **(right)**.

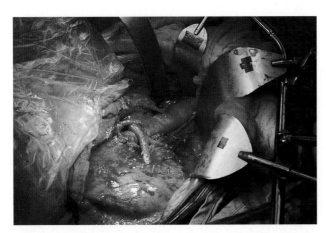

Figure 7-52. Operative photograph showing a self-retaining retraction system used to expose the distal thoracic and upper abdominal aorta after transabdominal medial visceral rotation.

Figure 7-50 demonstrates the superior and lateral limits of exposure through a midline incision when the route to the vessels has been a medial visceral rotation. The rotation and elevation of the left costal margin facilitate the view and ease of access without changing the limits. This is shown dramatically in the left panel of Fig. 7-51, where the costal margin is *in situ.* This is contrasted with the right panel of Fig. 7-51, where the division of costal margin and diaphragm allows extension of exposure into the chest by removal of the anatomic barrier. The operative photographs, Figs. 7-52 and 7-53, demonstrate the two exposures and the advantages for access, but not changes in limits, afforded by the use of self-retaining retractor systems. The sectors on view appended by a transabdominal and thoracoabdominal exposure of the upper aorta are shown in Fig. 7-54. Figure 7-55 is an operative photograph showing the sector of view obtained by a thoracoabdominal exposure.

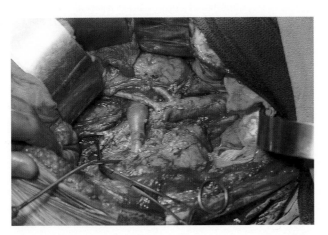

Figure 7-53. Operative photograph showing a thoracoabdominal medial visceral rotation approach to thoracoabdominal aorta and branches.

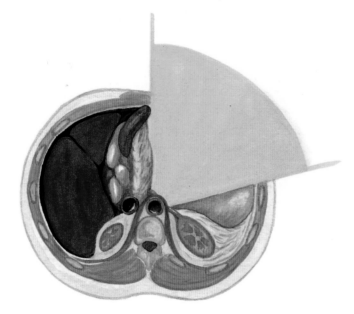

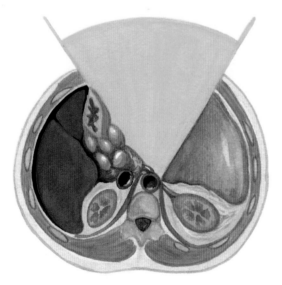

Figure 7-54. Cross-sectional views of the abdomen. The thoracoabdominal approach provides the sector of visibility shown at the **top**, whereas the transabdominal medial visceral rotation provides the sector of exposure and sight line as illustrated at the **bottom**.

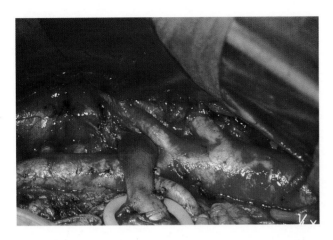

Figure 7-55. Operative photograph showing the lateral vector of a thoracoabdominal exposure. This represents the surgeon's line of sight.

ARTERIES OF THE TRUE AND FALSE PELVIS

The terminal common iliac artery and its branches can be well exposed through an extraperitoneal approach (Fig. 7-56). The skin incision is made obliquely in the iliac fossa halfway between the umbilicus and the anterior superior iliac spine, parallel to the inguinal ligaments. An incision of adequate length is required, generally about 20 to 25 cm. The subcutaneous tissue is divided in the line of the incision, and a muscle-splitting technique is then utilized to gain access to the extraperitoneal route to the vessel. Fibers of the external oblique muscle and aponeurosis are split in their line, and the external oblique muscle is retracted. The internal oblique muscle is then split in its line, and the fibers again are retracted, facilitating exposure of the transversus abdominis whose fibers run horizontally in the wound and are split along that line. Adequate retraction exposes the transversalis fascia and the underlying peritoneum. Then, after adequate wound retraction has been established, careful dissection is performed to create a cavity behind the transversalis fascia in the potential preperitoneal space. This dissection is continued inferiorly toward the iliac fossa. The plane lies between the peritoneum and, initially, the anterior abdominal wall, turning around onto the posterior abdominal wall until the psoas major muscle is clearly identified. The peritoneal sac can then be swept medially and upward to expose the anterior surface of psoas major and the major vessels of the iliac fossa. The vessels in this area are richly endowed with periarterial lymphatics, and careful attention should be directed to ligating major divided lymphatic trunks. The development of a lymphatic collection is one of the complications of wound healing in this area well recognized by the transplant surgeons, and the prevention of a major lymph leak facilitates complication-free healing after this exposure (Fig. 7-57).

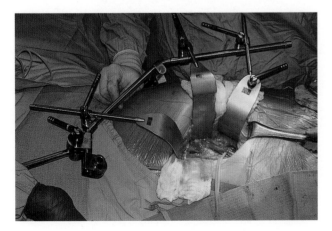

Figure 7-56. Operative photograph of self-retaining retractor used to provide right retroperitoneal exposure of the iliac vessels.

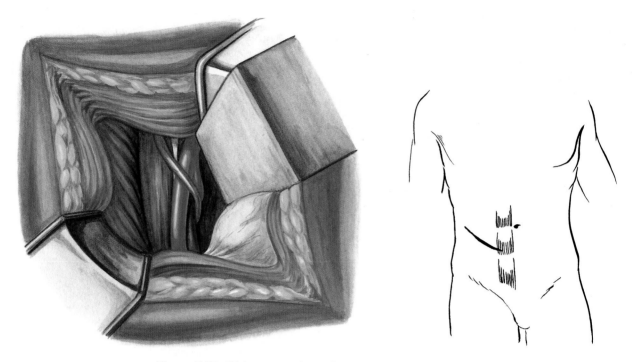

Figure 7-57. Right extraperitoneal exposure of the pelvic vessels.

This incision and route to the pelvic vessels provides excellent visualization and the ability to mobilize the whole of the external and internal iliac arteries to procure them as grafts or to deal with localized disease (Fig. 7-58).

Restoration

Restoration of this exposure is straightforward. The replacement of the peritoneal sac obliterates the submuscular dead space provided that attention has been paid to achieving hemostasis and that there is no lymph leak. If the deep wound is at all moist, a small suction drain should be placed before muscle closure. The muscles are reapproximated using absorbable suture material for the two inner layers. The aponeurosis of external oblique is closed with a running continuous suture of nonabsorbable mate-

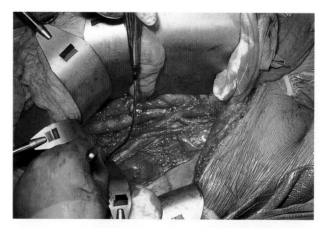

Figure 7-58. Operative photograph showing retroperitoneal exposure of the right iliac artery and its branches.

rial. Healing because of the muscle-splitting incision is rapid and secure with low risk of hernia formation. The skin is approximated.

The infrarenal abdominal aorta can be approached through an extraperitoneal route using an oblique incision placed in the flank to get access higher in the abdomen with the advantages of modern anesthesia, pain control, etc. However, little realistic benefit accrues to the patient with this approach compared with a formal transperitoneal route to the aortic segment.

EXPOSURE OF THE INFERIOR VENA CAVA

The exposure of the great veins within the abdomen has received little formal description in most textbooks of vascular surgery. However, the surgeon may be called on to expose the cava for the now rarely required caval ligation or to deal with trauma or tumor. Thus, an understanding of the best approaches and routes to these vessels is considered an integral part of the vascular surgeon's armamentarium.

Exposure of the Infrarenal Inferior Vena Cava

With modern anesthesia, the most expeditious exposure of the infrarenal inferior vena cava is a transabdominal approach. Adequate access to the cava can be obtained either through a long midline incision or through a transversely placed incision above the umbilicus. Once the abdomen is entered, the transverse colon is elevated out of the wound and surrounded by warm towels. The small bowel is identified and packed in a bowel bag and retracted to the right. The viscera are retained with splanchnic blades of the self-retaining retractor system.

The retroperitoneum is entered in the right side of the groove between the cava and the aorta, and the standard mobilization of the posterior peritoneum is performed, with the incision extended cephalad and dividing the attachments of the duodenum—the ligaments of Treitz. Once the duodenum is mobilized and retracted to the right, the incision can be carried superiorly into the base of the transverse mesocolon, thus exposing the inferior vena cava to above the levels of entry of the renal veins. The inferior vena cava can be mobilized circumferentially for whatever distance is required, and this approach also gives access to the whole of the iliac venous system and the body of the cava in its infrarenal extent.

The inferior vena cava overlies the right sympathetic trunk, and the circumferential mobilization of the vessel displays this structure, which should be protected. In order to fully mobilize the cava, the aorta itself may require at least partial mobilization on its right side in order to expose the requisite amounts of the cava.

Restoration

Standard restoration of the retroperitoneum, with approximation of the posterior peritoneum and standard closures of the abdominal wall, restore the anatomy.

Retroperitoneal Route to the Inferior Vena Cava

An alternative approach to the cava is the right retroperitoneal approach. A transverse incision extending from the tip of the ninth costal cartilage to about halfway across the anterior rectus sheath is used. The external oblique aponeurosis and the anterior sheath are divided, exposing the fleshy fibers of the internal oblique, which are divided in the line of the wound. The transversus abdominis muscle can be split along the line of its fibers. A mobilization of the peritoneum by developing the plane anteroinferiorly until psoas major is identified and then sweeping the peritoneum cephalad and to the left exposes the psoas major and quadratus lumborum in the base of the wound. The ureter is mobilized anteriorly with the peritoneum, and the only structure on display medial to the psoas major will be the inferior vena cava. Although this approach to the cava has been used for the placement of fenestrating clips in the past, the exposure generated is limited and imposes restricted access to the other intraabdominal organs.

Total Exposure of the Inferior Vena Cava by Right Medial Visceral Rotation

The whole of the right side of the retroperitoneum and the cava can be exposed by right-to-left medial viscera rotation. The patient is positioned supine, and access to the peritoneal cavity is obtained through a long midline incision or a transverse incision placed about the umbilicus (Fig. 7-59).

The right colon and cecum are mobilized by division of the lateral peritoneal attachments, and a plane between the colonic mesentery and the posteriorly placed kidney, adrenal gland, and ureter is developed similar to that on the left-hand side. The dissection is accomplished more easily on the right-hand side because of the greater mobility and ease of identification of the plane behind the right colon. An extensive Kocher maneuver of the duodenum, with division of its lateral superior and inferior attachments, allows the duodenum to be retracted to the left along with the head of pancreas and hepatic flexure. This maneuver allows visualization of the inferior vena cava throughout its whole length. The liver is rotated toward the left to facilitate exposure of the intrahepatic component. This is accomplished by division of the right triangular ligament and the peritoneal attachments to the bare area of the diaphragm. Once that maneuver has been accomplished, the cava can be seen from its commencement to its entry into the diaphragm at the level of T-8. Only one major structure is at serious risk during this mobilization, and that is the right ureter. The vena cava can be controlled and opened to allow for tumor or thrombus removal, and the caval wall can be resected and replaced if required (Fig. 7-60).

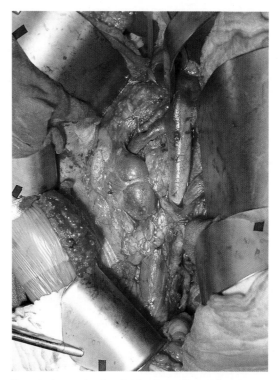

Figure 7-59. Operative photograph of a right retroperitoneal exposure of the inferior vena cava, renal vein, and kidney.

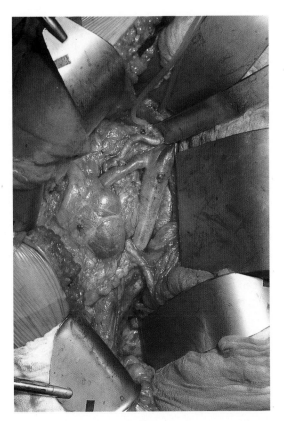

Figure 7-60. Operative photograph showing the inferior vena cava displaced and retracted at the pararenal level utilizing right-to-left medial visceral rotation.

Restoration

As on the left side, the conduct of the retroperitoneal dissection with the correct identification of the cleavage plane is the critical prerequisite for the restoration. Return of the viscera obliterates dead space and provides cover of viable tissue for the vascular wound. Standard closure of the abdominal wall completes the restoration.

Exposure of the Supraduodenal Vena Cava in the Posterior Wall of the Foramen of Winslow

The supraduodenal inferior vena cava is often best approached through a right sub-costal incision (Fig. 7-61). The patient is placed supine with a sandbag or table rest elevated beneath the lower right ribs and right hip. The skin incision is made from the midline obliquely to the level of the tenth costal cartilage, about 2 inches below and parallel to the costal margin. To permit additional exposure, this incision can be extended across the midline as an upper abdominal chevron. Aponeurotic and muscle fibers are divided in the line of the wound with division of the rectus abdominis muscle and posterior sheath allowing entry to the peritoneal cavity. The liver is retracted cephalad, and the transverse colon and hepatic flexure are retracted caudally. There is usually no need to mobilize the duodenum to gain satisfactory exposure of the infrahepatic cava. The retroperitoneum over the vena cava in the posterior wall of the foramen of Winslow is incised adjacent to the caudate lobe of the liver where it is at its thinnest. Once the vena cava wall is brought in view, the mobilization can continue up to the caudate lobe and as far inferiorly as the renal veins.

EXPOSURE OF THE PORTAL VEIN AND ITS MAJOR TRIBUTARIES

The portal vein lies in the free edge of the lesser omentum in the anterior wall of the foramen of Winslow (Fig. 7-62). It lies behind the common bile duct and the hepatic artery and is separated from the cava by the foramen. This part of the portal vein is best approached using the subcostal incision described above for the supraduodenal cava approach. The patient is positioned similarly. The free edge of the lesser omentum is identified, and the peritoneum over the posterolateral aspect of the free edge of the lesser omentum is incised. The common bile duct is identified, and the parietal peritoneal incision is carried along below the duct to expose the required length of vein. The duct is cleaned and retracted anteriorly with a small retractor, revealing the portal vein. The areolar coverings and the neural tissue surrounding the portal vein are incised, and the vein wall is clearly identified. The vein is mobilized using blunt and sharp dissection and is encircled by a rubber or plastic sling. Once control has been obtained, circumferential mobilization can continue cephalad and caudad to expose the required length of portal vein. The major risks during this dissection are the small medially placed pancreatic tributaries that must be ligated before division. These veins can represent a source of profuse blood loss in patients with portal hypertension if they are divided inadvertently. This dissection requires strict attention to the principles of scissors and forceps dissection and requires meticulous retraction and retention of the viscera.

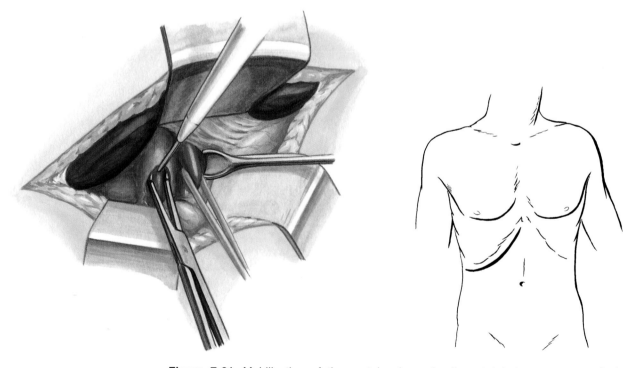

Figure 7-61. Mobilization of the portal vein and adjacent inferior vena cava (being exposed) through a subcostal incision with transabdominal route to the vessels.

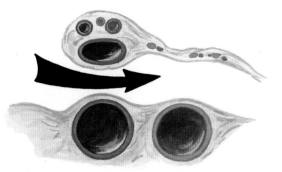

Figure 7-62. Cross section of the free edge of the lesser omentum. The *arrow* shows a space between the portal vein above and inferior vena cava below adjacent to the aorta in the retroperitoneum.

EXPOSURE OF THE SPLENIC VEIN

There are two available routes that can be used to expose the splenic vein. The first and simpler of these is the transperitoneal exposure. However, in patients with previously operated abdomens, other complications, or obliterated peritoneal cavities, a retroperitoneal approach is available.

The transabdominal approach is usually performed using a midline incision, or in some cases, a transverse incision across the epigastrium. Depending on the anatomy found at the time of abdominal exploration, the vein can be mobilized either from the infracolic compartment or may be accessed by dividing the gastrocolic ligaments and retracting the transverse colon downward. The self-retaining retractor system greatly facilities these difficult vascular exposures.

If an infracolic approach is used, the transverse colon is elevated out of the wound, and the small bowel packed off in a bag. The posterior peritoneum in the groove between the aorta and vena cava is opened, and a full mobilization of the fourth part of the duodenum and the duodenojejunal flexure is undertaken. The extension of the peritoneal division to the root of the transverse mesocolon allows exposure of the area of interest in the field. The left renal vein is mobilized circumferentially from its entry into the vena cava out toward the renal hilus. The structure at risk in this mobilization is the lumbar vein entering the proximal left renal vein posteriorly. Once the renal vein has been cleared, attention is turned to the substantial lymph nodes and lymphatic tissue that lie between the anterior border of the splenic vein and the renal vein. This lymph node mass and the associated neural tissue should be excised in order to facilitate exposure of the splenic vein. The mass is excised as far medially as the superior mesenteric artery. The pancreas is elevated by the retraction. The posterior surface, which is on clear view, is inspected, and the splenic vein is identified. The periadventitial coverings of the splenic vein are divided along the line of the vein on the posterior surface of the pancreas. Once an adequate length of the posterior surface of the vein has been exposed, depending on the reconstruction to be used, the groove between the pancreatic tissue and the splenic vein is developed to allow the application of the side-biting clamp and so obviate the need for complete mobilization of the vein from its bed, thus avoiding the fragile pancreatic tributaries.

If the route to the vessel is through the gastrocolic ligament, usually the falciform ligament is divided, and the gastrocolic ligament is divided on the gastric side of the gastroepiploic arcade from the pylorus to the short gastric vessels. The right gastroepiploic vessels are also divided near the pylorus. The peritoneum along the inferior border of the pancreas is divided, and the pancreas is mobilized from the superior mesenteric vein medially to the region of the tail in its lateral extent. Following that maneuver, the inferior border of the gland is rotated cephalad to expose the splenic vein in the posterior

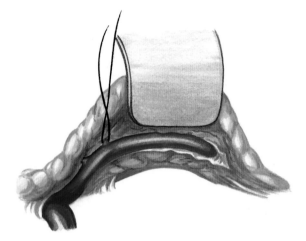

Figure 7-63. Elevated pancreas with the splenic vein and a tributary being controlled.

surface of the gland. The periadventitial tissue is incised, exposing the posterior aspect of the vein, and the vessel is exposed as far as the superior mesenteric vein and laterally as far as required to be able to perform the index operation.

An important aspect of preparation of the vein for a Warren shunt is that the initial mobilization of the splenic vein is undertaken near its junction with the superior mesenteric vein. The dissection around the circumference of the proximal splenic vein must always be performed under direct vision. This site is chosen because it is free of the troublesome posterior tributaries from the pancreas (Fig. 7-63). With the dilation of the vein during portal hypertension, the pancreatic tributaries are taken up into the wall, causing a foreshortening of the pancreatic tributaries and making their initial control more difficult. The inferior mesenteric vein should be divided. After the most proximal portion of the splenic vein has been circumferentially mobilized, the dissection proceeds carefully along the pancreatic aspect of the splenic vein. These small foreshortened venous tributaries must be ligated until a sufficient length of vein has been mobilized in continuity.

Restoration

Standard technique of restoration for the intraabdominal viscera are used to restore the anatomy after the completion of the index operation.

Retroperitoneal Exposure of the Splenic Vein

On occasion, because of difficulties within the peritoneal cavity, a retroperitoneal approach can be used to expose the splenic and renal veins. The patient is placed in a modified left lateral position, and a kidney rest on the table is elevated in order to facilitate the exposure.

The skin incision is placed beginning at the posterior axillary line in the 11th intercostal space and is carried anteriorly over the abdomen in that line onto the anterior abdominal wall. The muscles of the anterior abdominal wall as well as latissimus dorsi are divided in the line of the skin wound. The wound edges are retracted using a self-retaining retractor system, which greatly facilitates the conduct of this exposure.

A retroperitoneal plane in front of the kidney is developed. This approach makes use of the embryologically predetermined plane between the endodermally derived structures contained within the peritoneal cavity and the structures of the urogenital ridge, kidney, ureter, and adrenal gland and the mesodermal structures of the posterior wall.

As previously described, in the thoracoabdominal approach to the aorta and in medial visceral rotation, careful attention to the development of this plane behind the pancreas and in front of Gerota's fascia is absolutely critical to the outcome of the procedure. Pancreatic damage and pancreatitis can occur if the plane is too anterior, and bleeding occurs if the plane is too far posterior. Once the retroperitoneal space has been developed, the dissection extends to the limits of the aorta and the vena cava, as has been described for the other exposures.

The aim of the exposure is to display the renal and splenic veins as in the previously described transabdominal approach. The surgeon's perspective, however, is quite different. The hilus of the kidney is closest to the surgeon, and the renal vein is seen in the base of the wound heading downward and backward to cross the aorta and gain entry to the inferior vena cava. The body of the pancreas and its tail, held by the retractors with the splenic vein in its posterior surface, is immediately in front of the surgeon in the depths of the wound. The periadventitial tissue over the splenic vein is incised, and the posterior surface of the vein is cleaned for the required length. The groove between the splenic vein and pancreas is then developed on either side of the vein to allow the bulging of the vein in preparation for application of a clamp.

No attempt is made to circumferentially mobilize the vein using the retroperitoneal approach because the foreshortened fragile pancreatic tributaries are a cause of considerable bleeding.

Restoration

At the completion of the index procedure, the restoration is completed by allowing the peritoneal sac to fall back and occupy the space from which it was mobilized. The abdominal musculature can be closed in layers.

EXPOSURE OF THE SUPERIOR MESENTERIC VEIN IN THE ROOT OF THE MESENTERY

Occasionally the superior mesenteric vein requires exposure. After the bowel has been retracted toward the right, the superior mesenteric artery is identified coursing along the base of the mesentery. The retroperitoneal incision is placed immediately behind the artery, and the retroperitoneum is opened. The artery is retracted anteriorly, and the dissection proceeds to identify the superior mesenteric vein coursing to the right of the superior mesenteric artery. Further mobilization of the posterior surface of the artery allows an adequate length of superior mesenteric vein to be identified.

Restoration

Restoration of this wound is accomplished by direct suture closure of the peritoneum.

LEFT GASTRIC VEIN

The left gastric vein receives tributaries that drain both the anterior and posterior surfaces of the lesser curve of the stomach. The vein ascends parallel to the lower curve until it reaches the level of the esophagogastric junction, where it receives tributaries from the esophagus. The vein then curves downward passing behind the lesser sac to enter the splenic vein at the level of the superior border of the duodenum.

Access to the left gastric vein is obtained by division of the two layers of the lesser sac above the lower part of the lesser curve. Simple suture closure of the peritoneum effects the restoration.

8
Upper Extremity

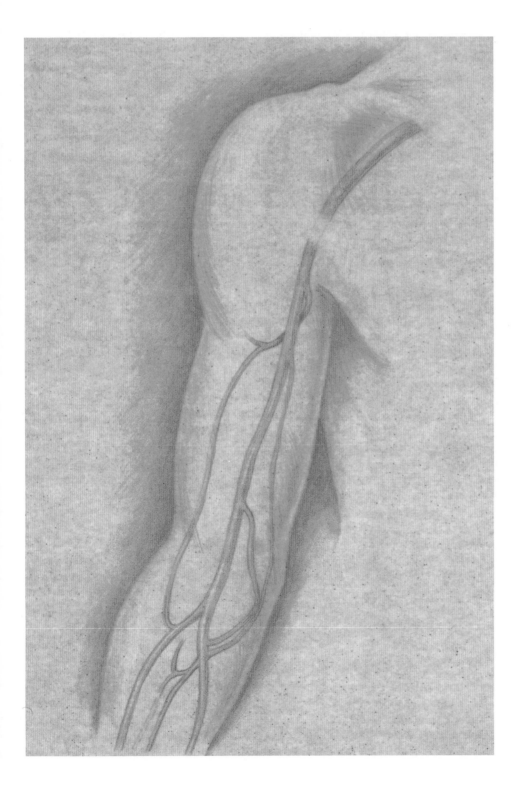

The arteries and veins of the upper extremity are superficially placed structures in the majority of cases. The facts that they are not deeply placed and that they have no viscera related to them make these vessels easily dissected and mobilized. The extent of tissue damage in their mobilization is minimal, with most exposures not requiring division of muscle fibers. The clear anatomic longitudinal relationships between the muscles and the neurovascular structures in the upper extremity similarly facilitate an easy, nontraumatic exposure of most of these vessels.

However, the vessels of the upper extremity are much less commonly operated on than those of the lower extremity, so review of the surgical anatomy is often required in planning any individual procedure.

SURGICAL ANATOMY

Subclavian Arteries

The anatomy of the subclavian artery has been described in the sections on the mediastinum **(Chapter 5)** and root of the neck **(Chapter 4)**. These vessels, which arise on the right side from the brachiocephalic artery and on the left from the aorta, leave the superior mediastinum behind the sternoclavicular joints. The vessels pass through the root of the neck, behind scalenus anterior muscle, and cross the first rib to enter the axilla.

Axillary Artery

The axillary artery begins as the continuation of the subclavian at the outer border of the first rib. It enters the axilla at the apex and passes across the first intercostal space to reach the lateral wall. The infraclavicular portion of the brachial plexus comes from above and behind the vascular plane to adopt the relationships that give the names to the cords of the plexus. The axillary vein lies medial and slightly below the artery.

Anteriorly, the artery is crossed by the pectoralis minor muscle as it passes to insert onto the coracoid process of the scapula. The tendon of the muscle divides the artery into its three parts, and it is the anatomic key to unlocking the exposure of the axillary artery.

In its course, the axillary artery lies on the origins of serratus anterior, the subscapularis muscle separated by the posterior cord of the brachial plexus. When it reaches the lateral wall of the axilla, it is related to the coracobrachialis muscle. In its third part, it lies on the tendon of latissimus dorsi and teres major.

The axillary artery changes its name to the brachial artery at the lower border of the teres major muscle. Once the artery emerges from under cover of the pectoralis major at the level of the anterior axillary fold, it and the brachial artery are covered superficially only by skin, subcutaneous tissue, and deep fascia of the arm from the axilla all the way to the elbow.

Brachial Artery

The brachial artery passes distally from its origin at the lower border of teres major to end at a bifurcation approximately 1 to 2 cm below the elbow joint. Throughout its course, the artery is easily palpable. Initially, the artery is felt in the groove between the coracobrachialis and biceps muscles, and then between the biceps and triceps muscle and, as the artery moves laterally, between biceps and brachialis. During its course, the vessel migrates from the medial side to the front of the arm, where it lies on the insertion of the coracobrachialis muscle and then the brachialis muscle. Eventually it passes in front of the biceps tendon.

At the front of the elbow, the bicipital aponeurosis crosses the artery, separating it from the median antecubital vein.

The profunda brachii artery is a large branch given off just after the beginning of the brachial artery itself. This artery follows the course of the radial nerve from its origin running backward between the long and medial heads of the triceps and then in the radial groove of the humerus, where it is covered by the lateral head of the triceps muscle.

Radial Artery

The radial artery is usually the smaller of the two branches of the brachial artery arising in the cubital fossa below the elbow joint. Like the brachial artery, whose general direction the radial artery follows, it is a very superficially placed vessel, being covered for most of its length by only skin, subcutaneous tissue, and deep fascia. The vessel passes along the medial side of the forearm to reach the front of the styloid process of the radius. In the forearm, the initial part of the artery is covered by the muscle belly of brachioradialis, but once the artery emerges from behind that muscle, it is superficial until it passes behind the flexor retinaculum. It then winds backward around the lateral side of the carpal bones, under cover of the tendons of abductor pollicis longus and the long and short extensors of the thumb, to reach the proximal space between the first and second metacarpal bones.

The radial artery, in its course down the forearm, lies on the biceps tendon supinator muscle, pronator teres, flexor digitorum superficialis, flexor pollicis longus, and pronator quadratus at the lower end of the radius.

The artery is most easily palpable just above the wrist, where it lies between the tendon of extensor pollicis longus and the lateral border of the radius.

The Ulnar Artery

The ulnar artery is usually larger than the radial. From the origin at the bifurcation of the brachial artery, the ulnar artery runs medially and downward to reach the medial side of the forearm about halfway between the wrist and elbow. It then runs downward to cross in front of the flexor retinaculum at the wrist and enters the hand to become the superficial palmar arch. In the forearm, the most important branch is the interosseous artery, which divides into anterior and posterior divisions, which descend in close proximity to the interosseous membrane.

Unlike the brachial and radial arteries, for the first two-thirds of its length the ulnar artery is covered by the muscle bellies of the forearm. As it crosses the forearm, it is covered by pronator teres, flexor carpi radialis, and the flexor digitorum superficialis. Then the artery lies between flexor digitorum superficialis and flexor carpi ulnaris. In the lower one-third of the forearm, it emerges from between the tendons of these two muscles and is then superficial, covered only by skin and fascia, until it passes behind palmaris brevis in the hypothenar eminence of the hand. During its course, the artery lies initially on the brachialis muscle then on flexor digitorum profundus.

Ulnar Nerve

The ulnar nerve has an interesting anatomic relationship to the vessels of the upper limb. The nerve, which begins from the medial cord of the brachial plexus, runs downward in the axilla to the medial side of the axillary artery between the artery and the axillary vein. It accompanies the brachial artery on its medial side to about the middle of the arm. Here the two structures diverge. The brachial artery inclines laterally and forward while the ulnar nerve pierces the medial intermuscular septum and passes medially and downward in the posterior muscular compartment in front of the medial head of the triceps. It passes through the ulnar groove on the medial epicodyle of the humerus to enter the forearm between the two heads of flexor carpi ulnaris. There it lies on the flexor digitorum profundus.

Just below the elbow, the ulnar artery and nerve are widely separated, but the lateral inclination of the ulnar artery and the downward course of the ulnar nerve bring the two structures together about one-third to one-half the way down the forearm. They travel together for the rest of their course, with the ulnar nerve always a medial relation to the artery and its venae comitantes.

Median Nerve

The median nerve has important relationships to the vessels in the arm and proximal forearm. It takes its origin from two of the cords of the brachial plexus, the lateral and medial cords. These two differing origins are closely related to the third part of the axillary artery, and they unite on the front or lateral side of the terminal part of the axillary artery. The median nerve accompanies the brachial artery throughout its whole course. Initially, it is placed on the lateral side of the artery. At about the junction of the upper third and lower two-thirds of the arm, at the level of the insertion of the coracobrachialis muscle, the nerve crosses the artery superficially to become a medial relation. It descends, in that relationship, with the brachial artery to the cubital fossa. It lies behind the aponeurosis of the biceps muscle and in front of the brachialis muscle. It enters the forearm between the two heads of pronator teres muscle.

It is a medial relation of the first $2^1/_2$ cm of the ulnar artery before it crosses in front of the ulnar artery from medial to lateral, separated from the artery by the ulnar head of pronator teres. For the rest of its course in the forearm, it has no direct relationship with the major axial vessels and is accompanied by a branch of the interosseous artery.

Radial Nerve

The radial nerve, derived from the posterior cord of the brachial plexus, is a posterior relation of the third part of the axillary artery and the proximal brachial artery. However, it rapidly loses this relationship as, accompanied by the profunda brachii, it winds backward in the radial groove of the humerus and is separated from the axial vessels. The radial nerve becomes associated with the radial artery only in the middle third of the forearm, where it lies behind the brachioradialis muscle to the lateral side of the radial artery. As it courses further down the forearm, it passes deep to the tendon of brachioradialis, winding around the lateral side of the radius to achieve, once again, the dorsal side of the limb.

Veins of the Upper Extremity

The named arteries of the forearm are accompanied by a pair of venae comitantes as the deep veins. Usually these coalesce into two veins that accompany the brachial artery. They transport the deep venous blood proximally until these two veins enter the single axillary vein at the lower margin of the subscapularis muscle.

The axillary vein, which is a continuation of the basilic vein, begins at the lower border of teres major. The vessel ascends through the axilla, is joined by the brachial veins, and, just before its termination, is joined by the cephalic vein coursing from the superficial tissues in the deltopectoral groove to enter the vein just below the clavicle. Above the lower border of the first rib, the axillary vein continues as the subclavian vein. This passes behind the clavicle, across the rib in front of the scalenus anterior muscle, to enter the root of the neck. The axillary vein lies medial to the artery and is separated in part from the artery by the medial pectoral nerve, the medial cord of the brachial plexus, the ulnar nerve, and the medial cutaneous nerve of the forearm. In the axilla, the axillary vein is joined by tributaries that accompany the major named arteries.

The upper limb has a specialized network of superficial veins. These veins frequently require access. They are the cephalic, basilic, and median veins of the forearm. All have extensive tributaries from the superficial venous network.

Cephalic Vein

The cephalic vein begins as a confluence of the radial part of the venous network of the dorsum of the hand and the lower dorsal surface of the forearm. It winds upward around the radial border of the forearm and ascends on the radial side of the anterior surface of the forearm. It receives numerous tributaries from the skin and superficial tissues from both surfaces of the forearm.

In front of the cubital fossa below the elbow, the cephalic vein gives off the median cubital vein, which crosses from lateral to medial, ascending to cross the joint line and join the basilic vein. During this course across the cubital fossa, the antecubital vein is joined posteriorly by a large communicating vein bringing blood from the deep veins of the forearm.

The cephalic vein continues to ascend through the arm lateral to the biceps. Just above the elbow, it is joined by the more laterally placed accessory cephalic vein. In the upper part of its course, it lies in and follows the deltopectoral groove. Below the clavicle, it passes behind the clavicular head of the pectoralis major and pierces the clavipectoral fascia to gain access to the terminal part of the axillary vein.

Basilic Vein

The basilic vein begins as the coalescence of the medial components of the dorsal venous network, and initially it runs proximally on the posterior surface of the forearm. It curves around the ulnar border a variable distance below the elbow to lie on the anterior surface of the forearm. From there, it ascends across the elbow joint and is joined by the median antecubital vein and continues proximally along the medial border of biceps. In this part of its course, it is a medial and superficial relation of the brachial artery and the medial cutaneous nerve of the forearm. About half-way up the arm, the basilic vein slides behind the deep fascia and continues its ascent on the medial side of the brachial artery to become the axillary vein.

Median Vein

The median vein of the forearm drains the much smaller palmar venous plexus. It begins in front of the wrist and ascends to the cubital fossa, where it joins either the antecubital vein or the basilic vein.

BASE OF NECK TO AXILLA: A TRANSITION ZONE

The nerves of the brachial plexus and the arteries ascending out of the chest come together as they cross the first rib behind the clavicle. These arterial and nervous structures pass between the scalene muscles with scalenus anterior in front and the medius/posterior complex behind. The structures enter the apex of the axilla to supply the arm. The venous structures are placed more anteriorly. The axillary vein crosses the first rib anterior to scalenus anterior muscle and occupies the space between the first rib and the clavicle. The relationships are shown in Fig. 8-2.

We are beginning to appreciate more pathology related to the anatomic relationships of axillary–subclavian veins. In order to expose this structure adequately at its site of transition, two incisions are required (Fig. 8-3). These incisions, placed above and below the clavicle, allow the safe and complete mobilization of the vein.

Our current understanding of compressive symptoms of the arterial and neural structures in the thoracic outlet syndrome indicates that most patients do not require first rib

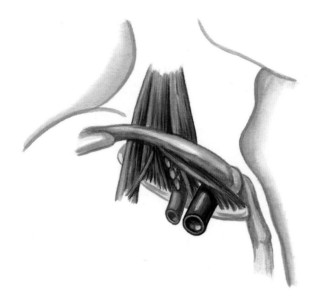

Figure 8-2. Apex of the axilla with its neurovascular and muscular structures.

resection. However, when there is compression of the vein, it always requires first rib removal for adequate correction. The exposure is well seen in Figs. 8-4 and 8-5.

This exposure exemplifies an approach consistent with our original stated thesis. The wound is engineered to create an optimum healing environment once the initiating and perpetuating cause of the problem has been removed. This is also a prime example of limits on exposure imposed by anatomic constraints, the problem being solved by using discontinuous approaches to obtain the required exposure.

Exposure of the Axillary Artery

The patient is positioned supine. The anterior chest, shoulder, and arm as far as the elbow should be prepared and included in the sterile field. The skin incision is placed below and parallel to the clavicle and is centered on the midpoint of that bone (Fig. 8-6). The incision is deepened through the superficial tissues and the fascia over the pec-

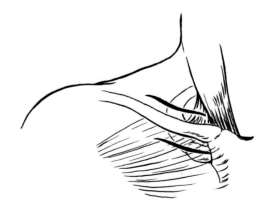

Figure 8-3. Supraclavicular and infraclavicular incisions used to create exposure for the subclavian vein.

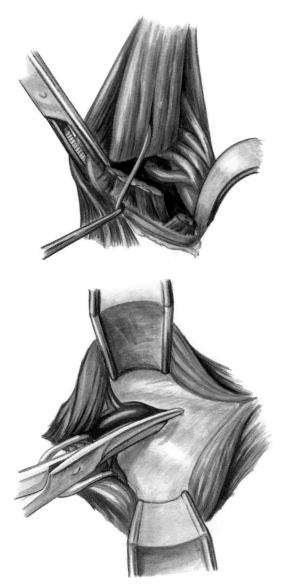

Figure 8-4. Lateral view of the scalene space with the middle scalene muscle transected and the anterior scalene muscle resected. The long thoracic nerve is being gently retracted laterally.

Figure 8-5. Pectoralis muscle fibers being separated and exposure of the subclavian vein.

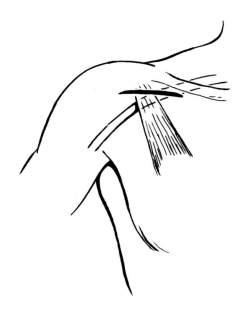

Figure 8-6. The infraclavicular skin incision.

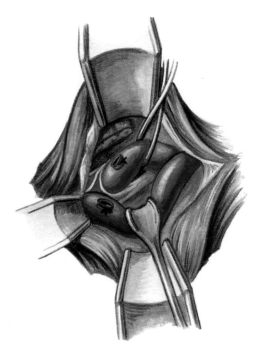

Figure 8-7. Proximal axillary artery and vein. The pectoralis minor has been divided.

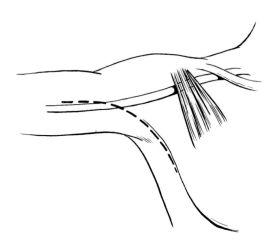

Figure 8-8. Proposed skin incision (*dotted line*) for exposure of the axillary and proximal brachial artery.

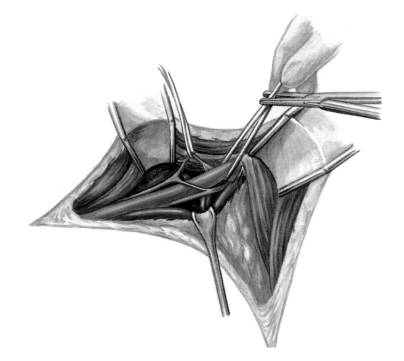

Figure 8-9. Exposure of the distal axillary and proximal brachial artery and vein. The pectoralis major is retracted rather than divided in this exposure.

toralis major muscle to expose the muscle fibers. The skin wound is held separated by a self-retaining retractor. The pectoralis major muscle is split in the line of the fibers between the clavicular and sternal heads of the muscle. The muscle fibers are split for the entire length of the wound and are retained apart by the self-retaining retractor system. The small modified wishbone system gives excellent retention of the muscle.

In the base of the wound, the pectoralis minor muscle will be seen coursing obliquely from below upward. The tendon of the muscle is identified and mobilized. The tendon is then divided close to the insertion into the coracoid process. The contraction of the pectoralis minor withdraws the tendon inferomedially and exposes the axillary vessels and brachial plexus.

The axillary vein is anteromedial and below the artery. It is easily dissected and retracted inferiorly if required. The periarterial tissue around the axillary artery is incised in the line of the vessel to reach the true periadventitial plane, and the artery is mobilized circumferentially for the distance required (Fig. 8-7).

Restoration

This exposure creates dead space. The area of division and retraction of the pectoralis minor is not repaired after the index operation. Indeed, if a tunnel is to be made from the axilla to the groin, the origin of that will be lateral to the pectoralis minor behind the pectoralis major muscle, creating a natural funnel into which will drain the inevitable fluid collection that occurs in the upper compartment of the conjoint wound. Suction drainage of this wound is mandatory after hemostasis has been secured to prevent the accumulation of fluid and subsequent tracking along the tunnel that is inevitable from the creation of the dead space.

Exposures of the Brachial Artery

1. Proximal brachial. On occasion it is necessary to extend the exposure of the axillary artery to the brachial (Fig. 8-8). This is achieved by extending the infraclavicular incision laterally to the deltopectoral groove and dividing the pectoralis major muscle (Figs. 8-9 and 8-10).

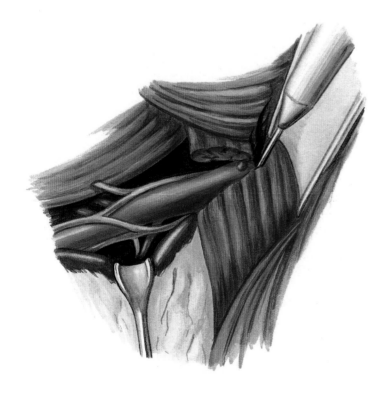

Figure 8-10. The axillobrachial region close up. The pectoralis minor muscle is being divided with electrocautery.

2. In the arm (Fig. 8-11). The brachial artery may be exposed in any part of its length in the arm by a simple skin incision placed over the vessel and dividing the superficial tissues and investing fascia of the arm. The artery is then immediately on display and can be circumferentially mobilized.

3. Above the elbow (Fig. 8-12). The brachial artery is usually exposed through a transverse incision placed above the elbow crease in the cubital fossa or a longi-

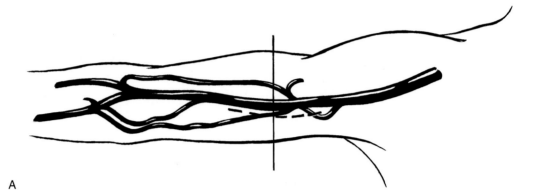

A

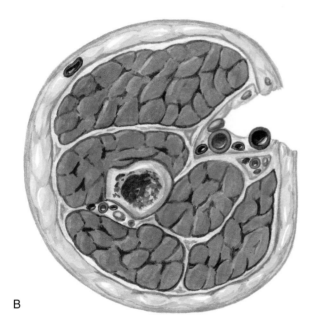

B

Figure 8-11. A: Line of a transverse view through the midarm. *Dotted line* depicts course of incision. **B:** Cross section of the arm showing the incision exposing the artery and vein. **C:** Longitudinal view through the midarm showing the brachial and basilic vein exposed.

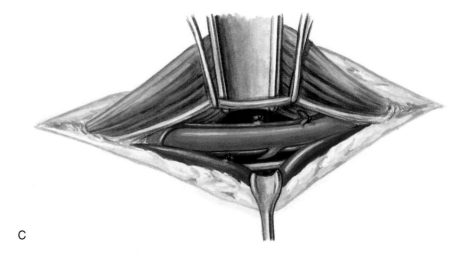

C

tudinal incision along the line of the vessel. A small 2-inch wound is made, centered on the arterial pulse. This is deepened through the subcutaneous tissue, and the fascia is incised. The brachial artery is seen coursing downward to pass behind the bicipital aponeurosis, which can be divided if required to provide further access. The vessel is readily mobilized from the accompanying structures by careful scissors and forceps dissection.

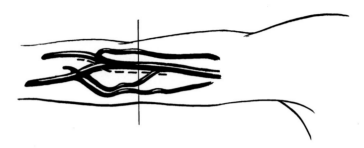

A

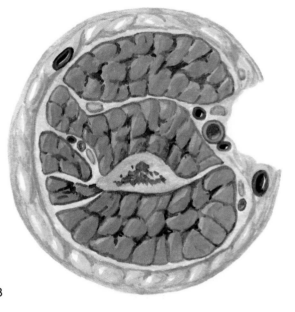

B

Figure 8-12. A: Proposed level of a cross section of the distal portion of the arm. **B:** Cross section of the arm showing the incision (*dotted line*) used to expose the brachial artery. **C:** Longitudinal exposure of the distal brachial artery.

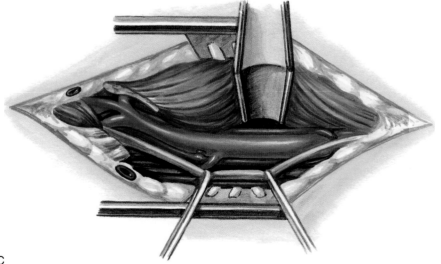

C

4. Below the elbow (Fig. 8-13). Below the elbow, the artery is covered by the variations of the cephalic and antecubital veins, which must be mobilized to allow access.

Exposure of the Radial Artery

The radial artery is easily exposed throughout its entire course in the forearm. However, it is usually required to be exposed only at the wrist (Fig. 8-14). In this location, it is very superficial and exposed by division of the skin and overlying tissues. The radial artery is, however, very liable to spasm, and before the artery is mobilized, the well-visualized radial sheath, in reality the deep fascia, is infiltrated with papaverine, which spreads longitudinally along that vessel. The sheath can then be opened and the artery mobilized by careful scissors and forceps dissection.

Restoration of all of these superficial wounds is by absorbable suture closure of the fascia and approximation of the skin. If the pectoralis major is divided in the proximal brachial exposure, it is reconstituted with absorbable sutures before fascial and skin closure.

Exposure of the Ulnar Artery

Exposure of the ulnar artery in its superficial part is obtained by skin and subcutaneous incision over the course of the vessel. Infiltration of the less well developed sheath and circumferential mobilization of the vessel are all that is required. This wound requires restoration, as has been described for the radial artery.

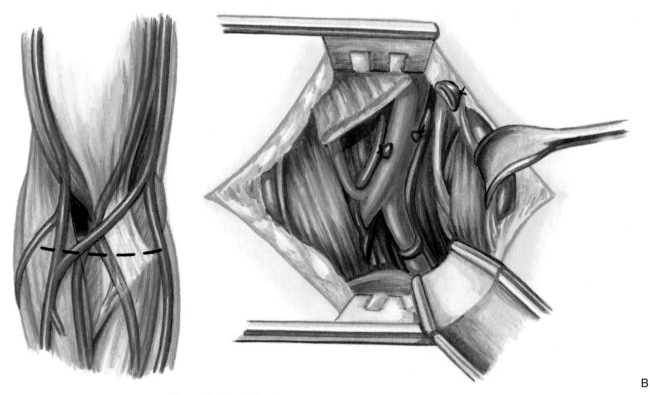

A

B

Figure 8-13. A: Surface anatomy of the lower aspect of the elbow region. Transverse skin incision is shown as a *dotted line.* **B:** Exposure of the brachial artery bifurcation.

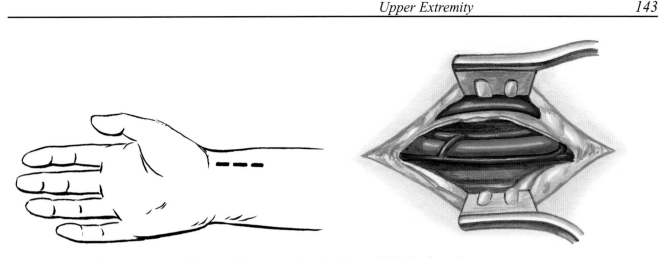

A   B

Figure 8-14. A: Site of exposure of the radial artery at the wrist (*dotted line*). **B:** Operative exposure through this wrist incision showing the cephalic vein and radial artery.

If it is required, the lower half to two-thirds of the artery can be exposed higher in the forearm by splitting the tissue between flexor carpi radialis and flexor digitorum superficialis.

Venous Exposures in the Upper Extremity

Superficial veins of the arm may all be accessed by skin incisions and a superficial wound placed immediately over the required access site. By placing the skin incision between the radial artery and cephalic vein at the wrist and creating small skin flaps, both of these vessels may be accessed through a single wound. Useful sites of venous access in the upper limb are at the wrist, back of the forearm, and the cephalic vein in the deltopectoral groove.

Large veins suitable for graft or graft implantation are readily accessible in the antecubital fossa. An incision placed transversely (Fig. 8-13) 2 cm below the elbow crease allows the rapid mobilization of the antecubital vein and all of its tributaries and ramifications, including the communicating vein on its posterior surface. The skin and superficial fascia are divided, and the appropriate length of vein mobilized, by careful scissors and forceps dissection. This wound is often the recipient end of the tunnel in arteriovenous graft placement, but because it can be restored without leaving dead space, no drains are required, and the superficial tissues can be closed with an absorbable suture and the skin approximated.

9

Lower Extremity

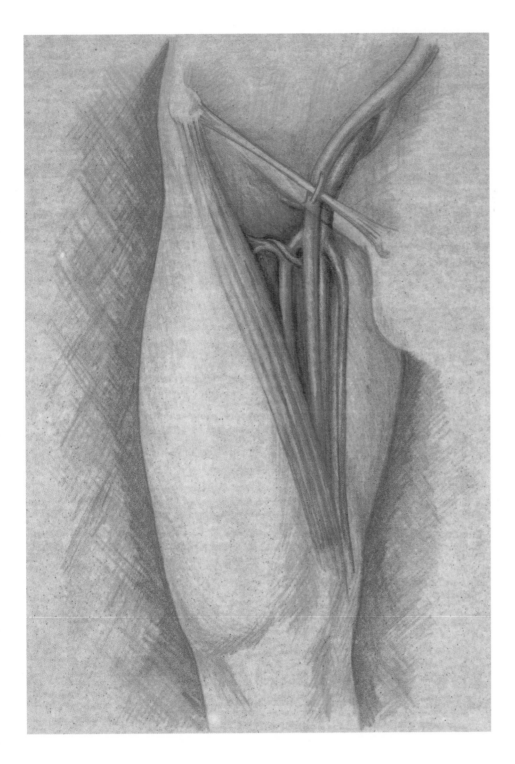

The vessels of the lower extremity are those most affected by atherosclerosis, and on a worldwide basis, they are those most approached by vascular surgeons. In **Chapter 2** we discussed the anatomy of the common femoral artery and its major branches and used that region to illustrate in practical terms the principles developed in **Chapter 1**. For completeness, the anatomy of these vessels is reproduced here.

SURGICAL ANATOMY OF THE COMMON FEMORAL ARTERY AND ITS MAJOR BRANCHES

The common femoral artery is the continuation of the external iliac artery and begins at the bifurcation of the common iliac artery at about the brim of the true pelvis. It runs downward and laterally along the medial border of the psoas major muscle, separated from the muscle by the iliac fascia. In front of the vessel and medially, there is a direct relationship of the artery to the parietal peritoneum, extraperitoneal fat, and the other extraperitoneal tissues. In addition, there are numerous lymph nodes and abundant lymph channels, which may cause troublesome lymph leaks after mobilization of structures in this area and require serious consideration by the surgeon when constructing a retroperitoneal tunnel. The vessel has no major branches until its termination, where the inferior epigastric and the deep circumflex iliac arteries are given off. Above these two branches, the external iliac artery is crossed by the lateral circumflex iliac vein, "the vein of sorrow," shortly before that vein enters into the external iliac vein.

Anatomically the common femoral artery begins behind the inguinal ligament and enters the femoral triangle at about the midpoint of its base. The vessel divides within the triangle to form the superficial femoral and profunda femoris arteries. The superficial femoral artery crosses the triangle and exits through the apex to enter the subsartorial canal. In life the femoral triangle corresponds to the depression below the groin crease (see the frontispiece on page 145). The triangle is formed by the inguinal ligament above the medial border of sartorius muscle and the medial border of adductor longus muscle. The floor of the triangle, which has a trough or gutter shape, is formed from above down and from lateral to medial by four muscles: iliacus, psoas major, pectineus, and adductor longus. The common femoral artery is related posteriorly to the psoas and pectineus muscles (Fig. 9-2).

The common femoral artery is enclosed for the first few centimeters of its length within the femoral sheath, a fascial condensation and inferior extension of the iliac fascia posteriorly and the transversalis fascia anteriorly. It is usually thought of as having, from lateral to medial, three compartments: an arterial compartment containing the femoral artery and the femoral branch of the genitofemoral nerve; a venous compartment containing the femoral vein; and the potential space called the femoral canal, which contains fat and the lymph node of Cloquet. The sheath is well developed and readily separated over the proximal common femoral artery, but it blends with the periarterial tissue toward and beyond the bifurcation of the common femoral artery.

The common femoral artery branches into two major vessels. The superficial femoral artery is usually the larger of the two branches and is the arterial conduit that carries blood to the leg. The profunda femoris artery is the artery of supply to the tissues of the thigh.

The superficial femoral artery passes through the femoral triangle and exits into the subsartorial canal by passing through the musculofascial apex of the femoral triangle (Fig. 9-3). This canal extends from the apex of the femoral triangle to the adductor hiatus in adductor magnus muscle, through which it gains access to the popliteal space and becomes the popliteal artery. The subsartorial space appears somewhat triangular when the thigh is seen in cross section, and it is bordered by the sartorius muscle medially, the vastus medialis anterolaterally, and the adductor muscles posteriorly—initially adductor longus and subsequently adductor magnus.

The profunda femoris artery arises from the posterolateral aspect of the common femoral. The medial and lateral circumflex femoral vessels are given off as branches soon after its origin, although in about 20% of patients these vessels arise from the

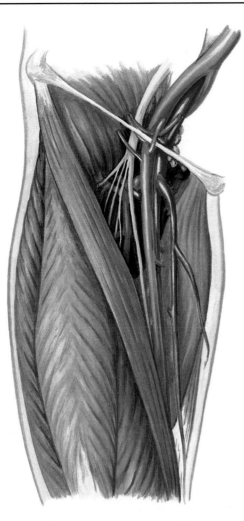

Figure 9-2. Neurovascular anatomy of the anteromedial thigh.

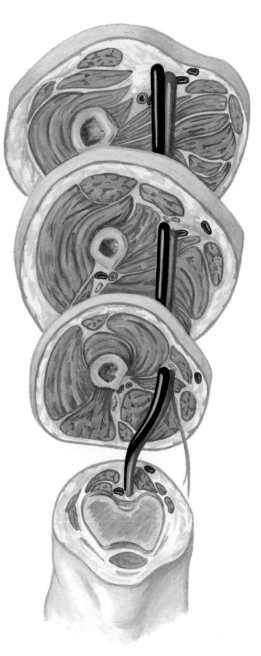

Figure 9-3. Four levels of the cross-sectional anatomy of the thigh.

common femoral artery at the level of the bifurcation. These arteries are important collaterals that can function in either direction, serving as reentry vessels from the cruciate anastomosis around the hip when the external iliac artery is stenotic or occluded or as supplying vessels to the cruciate anastomosis when the internal iliac artery is severely diseased. The lateral circumflex femoral branch has ascending and descending branches, the latter of which runs along the vastus lateralis to the knee.

The profunda femoris artery usually has three perforating arteries that supply the musculature of the thigh and the profunda ends by piercing adductor magnus in what is sometimes called the fourth perforating branch. The first perforating artery has an ascending and descending branch, and the other perforating vessels are connected by a rich anastomotic network. In addition to the perforating branches, there are several large muscular branches that anastomose in the medial compartment in the thigh to form a series of anastomotic vessels that are parallel to the perforators. At the lower end of the artery, the medial collateral branches anastomose with popliteal muscular branches, particularly the medial superior geniculate artery. The lateral collateral pathway anastomoses with the lateral superior geniculate muscular branches. Through the geniculate system around the knee joint, these profunda branches carry blood to the tibial recurrent and upper muscular branches of the main crural arteries when the popliteal artery is occluded. Thus, the profunda femoris collateral system has the capacity to bring blood from the cruciate anastomosis around the hip joint to the tibial vessels.

Shortly after the bifurcation of the common femoral artery, the profunda femoris artery passes behind the lateral border of adductor longus and is covered by that muscle. Posteriorly the artery lies from above to below on pectineus muscle, adductor brevis, and adductor magnus.

Immediately below the bifurcation of the common femoral artery, the profunda femoris is crossed by the lateral circumflex femoral vein just before that major tributary enters the common femoral vein.

Within the femoral triangle, the common femoral artery and its bifurcation are surrounded by lymph channels, and above the femoral sheath and deep to the fascia lata, the deep inguinal nodes are found medial to the common femoral vein. Above the fascia lata, the superficial nodes, which run lateral to where the main trunk of the saphenous vein enters the fossa ovalis, are an immediate anterior relation of the artery and are at risk of injury during the incision and development of the route of access to the artery. These nodes are contained in the superficial fascia, which, in the region of the groin, has a well-developed membranous layer. The superficial fascia of the groin is referred to as Camper's fascia.

The anatomy of the groin region determines the method of exposure of the common femoral vessels, the route of access to the arteries, and the closure required to conform to principles we have previously set forth. In addition, the anatomy dictates how and where the tunnels entering and leaving this region should be begun or ended.

The superficial femoral artery descending under cover of sartorius in Hunter's canal eventually passes through the opening in adductor magnus to enter the popliteal fossa to become the popliteal artery.

Popliteal Artery

The popliteal fossa is a very important transitional area in the anatomy of the lower extremity (Fig. 9-4). Because of the movements of the knee, all of the structures passing from the thigh to the leg must traverse the space. The space must be filled with tissue with a consistency that can offer cushioning protection to the structures and yet be able to move and change shape to accommodate the 150° range of motion possible at the joint. This is also important because the popliteal space represents the area where the major axial nerves, which have descended in the posterior thigh, become realigned with the more anterior traveling vessels. These structures are then intimately associated for the rest of their course.

The popliteal fossa is located behind the knee and is an elongated diamond-shaped space in which the points of the diamond are rounded (Fig. 9-5). In front it is bounded

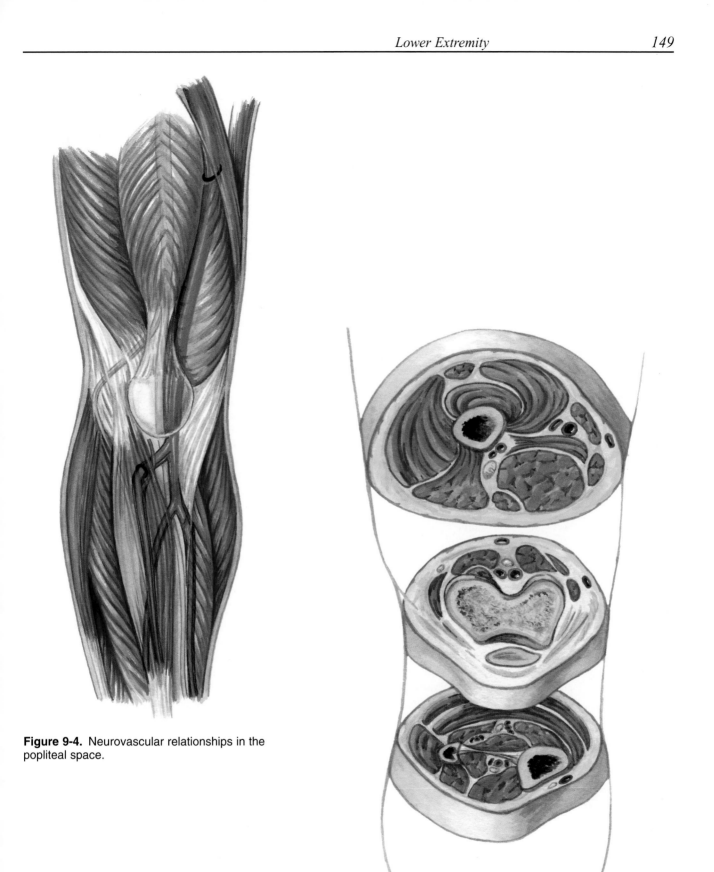

Figure 9-4. Neurovascular relationships in the popliteal space.

Figure 9-5. Cross sections through the proximal and distal popliteal regions.

by the back of the lower part of the femur and the upper part of the tibia, the capsule of the knee joint, and, below that, by the popliteus muscle. Posteriorly the boundaries are the investing fascia, subcutaneous tissue, and skin. Its posterolateral margins are made up of the biceps femoris muscle and tendon above and by the lateral head of the gastrocnemius inferiorly. Posteromedially the other two hamstring muscles, semitendinosus and semimembranosus, form the superior part of the border, and inferiorly the medial head of gastrocnemius completes the boundaries of the fossa.

Because of the bulk of the muscular tendinous borders, the posterior wall of the fossa is less than 2.5 cm wide, and the contents are thus almost completely covered. The superficial part of the fossa transmits the short saphenous vein to about the level of the knee joint. In addition, the posterior femoral cutaneous nerve is found superficially.

The popliteal artery occupies space on the floor of the fossa. Initially it travels downward and slightly laterally from the adductor hiatus and then passes directly down the popliteal space from between the condyles of the femur to the lower border of the popliteus muscle. From there, it divides into the anterior tibial and the tibioperoneal trunk.

The popliteal vein, which may be double, is formed by the junction of the anterior and posterior tibial veins at the lower border of the popliteus muscle. It is closely bound to the popliteal artery by thicker than normal areolar tissue, which forms a "pseudosheath" around the two structures in the fossa. This close attachment of artery, vein, and, in the smaller vessels, the artery and venae comitantes is a feature of the anatomy of the lower popliteal, tibioperoneal trunk, and proximal crural vessels.

At its origin the vein is posteromedial to the artery, but as it ascends, it becomes posteriorly placed between the heads of the gastrocnemius. Above the level of the knee joint, it is posterolateral, but it assumes an almost true lateral relationship by the time it reaches the adductor hiatus. In the fossa, the popliteal vein receives the short saphenous vein and the veins that accompany the named branches the popliteal artery.

The other major structures in the popliteal space are the distal continuations of the sciatic nerve, the tibial and common peroneal nerves. These nerves enter the popliteal space through the apex of the fossa. The nerves travel through the lower part of the thigh, lying on adductor magnus and covered by the long head of the biceps femoris muscle. They enter the popliteal space in a plane well posterior to the vessels, and the nerves are separated from the vessels initially by fat.

The tibial nerve crosses behind the vessels from lateral to medial and becomes closely associated with the distal popliteal and tibioperoneal trunk before leaving the space in front of the arch of the origin of soleus muscle in company with the tibioperoneal trunk.

The common peroneal nerve remains closely applied to the medial margin of the biceps femoris muscle and tendon and thus descends on the lateral side of the fossa to the head of the fibula. There it lies between the tendon of the biceps muscle and the lateral head of the gastrocnemius muscle. It passes around the neck of the fibula deep to the peroneus longus muscle to reach the peroneal compartment, where it forms the superficial and deep peroneal nerves.

The popliteal space contains lymph nodes, and the remainder of it is filled with loculated fat.

In order to facilitate exposures of the vessels in the region, it is sometimes necessary to divide muscular structures on the medial side of the leg and thigh. Thus, a brief review of the anatomy of the muscles subject to division is appropriate.

Muscles of the Region

Semitendinosus

The semitendinosus muscle arises from the tuberosity of the ischium, sharing a common tendon with the long head of the biceps femoris. It also arises from an aponeurosis between the two muscles that continues for a short distance after their origin. The fibers run downward to insert by a long tendon, which begins in the midthigh and lies on the surface of the semimembranosus muscle to the upper medial surface of the shaft of the tibia. This insertion lies behind that of sartorius and is below the gracilis insertion.

Semimembranosus

The semimembranosus muscle arises from a thick tendon on the ischial tuberosity and from a large membranous tendon/aponeurosis to form a large muscle that converges into a complicated tendon of insertion. At the level of the knee joint, it divides into various components that attach principally to the medial condyle of the tibia and to adjacent bone.

Gracilis

The gracilis muscle is placed superficially on the medial side of the thigh. It arises from the body of the pubis, the inferior ramus of the pubis, and part of the adjacent ischial ramus. Thus, the origin of the muscle is very broad. The muscle tapers to a tendon after running vertically down the thigh. The tendon passes across the condyle of the femur posterior to the tendon of sartorius and is inserted into the upper part of the shaft of the tibia below the tibial condyle between the insertions of semimembranosus and sartorius.

Sartorius

The sartorius muscle is the longest muscle in man. It arises from the anterior superior iliac spine and the adjacent bone on the front of the iliac bone below the spine. The muscle crosses the anterior thigh from lateral to medial, and, on the medial side, it descends almost vertically to insert though a tendon and aponeurosis into the upper part of the medial surface of the tibia immediately in front of the insertion of gracilis and semitendinosis muscles.

Gastrocnemius

The gastrocnemius muscle arises by two heads from each of the condyles of the femur. The medial head, which is the larger of the two, arises from the upper and posterior part of the medial condyle behind the adductor tubercle and from the popliteal surface of the femur just above the condyle. The lateral head arises from the lateral condyle and the immediate supracondylar surface of the femur. Both of the heads take some slips of origin from the immediately adjacent part of the joint capsule. These origins are continued on the posterior surface of the muscle as a tendinous expansion from which the muscle fibers arise. The fibers then merge into a broad aponeurosis that develops on the anterior surface of the muscles. The anterior aponeurosis converges and merges with the tendon of soleus to become the Achilles tendon.

Soleus

The soleus muscle is placed deeply behind the gastrocnemius. It arises from the soleal line and middle third of the medial border of the tibia. It gains a fibular origin from the back of the head and upper quarter of the shaft. Stretching between the medial and lateral bony origins is the soleal arch. This strong fibrous arch is found at the level of the lower part of the popliteus muscle, and beneath it pass the axial structures leaving the popliteal fossa. Because of the anatomic arrangements as these structures pass beneath the soleal arch, they lie on the deep muscle group of the calf. The origin of soleus from the arch is aponeurotic with most of the muscle fibers arising from the posterior surface of the aponeurosis. The muscle passes downward and becomes tendinous, with the tendon converging and merging with the tendon of gastrocnemius to form the Achilles tendon.

The deep group of muscles in the calf—the popliteus, flexor hallucis longus, flexor digitorum longus, and tibialis posterior—form the muscular carpet on which the axial nervous and vascular structures traverse the leg.

Branches of the Popliteal Artery

The branches the popliteal artery are important anatomically because they supply end arteries to the soleus and gastrocnemius muscles and form the major collateral arcade around the knee joint.

The sural arteries are usually two small straight arteries that supply the muscle. They arise from the posterior surface of the popliteal artery and diverge from it above or at the level of the knee joint.

The major collateral network is formed largely by the geniculate arteries. This is usually described as having three major contributions. First, a supreme geniculate, which is unpaired, usually arises from the medial side of the popliteal artery. Paired superior geniculate arteries arise from the medial and lateral side of the vessel at the level of the top of the femoral condyles, and a pair of inferior geniculate arteries arise from the popliteal artery under the heads of the gastrocnemius muscle.

These five major vessels contribute to the deep and superficial arterial anastomotic vessels around the knee. The network is also contributed to from the major crural vessels by the anterior and posterior tibial recurrent arteries ascending from those arteries in the calf toward the knee.

Crural Vessels

Anterior Tibial Artery

The anterior tibial artery is the smaller of the two terminal branches of the popliteal artery and arises from its parent at the lower border of the popliteus muscle. It passes forward between the origins of tibialis posterior muscle and penetrates the interosseous membrane to enter the anterior compartment of the leg. During that part of its course, it is medial to the neck of the fibula.

The vessel then turns downward and runs inferiorly. For about two-thirds of its length, it lies on the interosseous membrane, and in the lower one-third of its course, it lies on the front of the tibia and the front of the ankle joint. The artery passes behind the extensor retinaculum and is continued in the foot as the dorsalis pedis artery. The artery is accompanied in its course by a pair of deep veins, the venae comitantes.

The deep peroneal nerve joins the artery soon after it enters the anterior compartment and runs with it through the leg. Initially the nerve, which had wound around the neck of the fibula from the popliteal space, is lateral to the artery, but from about the middle of the leg, it has a somewhat variable anterolateral relationship with the vessel. The initial one-third of the artery lies between tibialis anterior and extensor digitorum longus. The artery's second third lies between tibialis anterior and extensor hallucis longus. In the final one-third of its course, it is covered only by skin, fascia, and the extensor retinaculum. At the level of the ankle joint, the laterally placed tendon of extensor hallucis longus crosses in front of the anterior tibial artery to become medial to it. The dorsalis pedis artery, the continuation of the anterior tibial, has its pulse easily palpated on the dorsum of the foot in the groove lateral to the tendon of extensor hallucis longus. Here it is very superficially placed, covered only by skin and fascia.

Tibioperoneal Trunk

The tibioperoneal trunk is the direct continuation of the popliteal artery as it passes behind the soleal arch. The vessel is of variable length, ranging from 0 to 5 cm before it bifurcates to form the posterior tibial and peroneal arteries. The tibioperoneal trunk lies on the tibialis posterior and is covered by gastrocnemius and soleus. It has an intimate relationship with a complex, thin-walled venous network that is closely adherent to the artery and may cause troublesome bleeding during its dissection. The tibioperoneal trunk is accompanied below the soleal arch and for its whole course by the tibial nerve.

Posterior Tibial Artery

This is the direct inferior continuation of the tibioperoneal trunk. It runs downward on the tibialis posterior muscle for much of its course, and in the lower part near the ankle, it lies on flexor digitorum longus, then on the tibia and back of the ankle joint. The artery passes posterior to the medial malleolus and divides to form the plantar arteries.

In the upper part, the artery is covered by gastrocnemius and soleus, whereas inferiorly it runs about $2^{1}/_{2}$ cm in front of the Achilles tendon and is covered only by skin and fascia before passing behind the flexor retinaculum and the abductor hallucis muscle.

A pair of deep veins accompany the artery as venae comitantes, and the posterior tibial nerve is a constant companion in the neurovascular bundle, as a medial relation at first and, in the lower part of the leg, as a posterior relation of the artery.

The Peroneal Artery

The peroneal artery passes from its origin obliquely laterally and downward toward the fibula. When it reaches the medial crest of the fibula, it descends vertically in a well-formed fibrous canal between flexor hallucis longus and tibialis posterior. On occasion, however, the artery runs in the substance of the flexor hallucis muscle. When viewed on an arteriogram in an anteroposterior projection, the peroneal artery runs downward in the middle of the leg to divide into anterior and posterior calcaneal branches above the ankle joint.

The peroneal artery has a pair of accompanying deep veins but has no major nerve traveling with it.

The Veins of the Lower Extremity

The veins of the lower extremity are divided into two major groups: the superficial and deep veins. The deep veins are further divided into three subsets. The first of these, the axial veins, are those that accompany the arteries of the same names. The veins, which are larger and accompany the more major arteries—the common femoral vein, the superficial femoral vein, and the profunda and popliteal veins—are usually single venous structures. However, the veins accompanying the smaller arteries, particularly those in the leg, achieve greater hemodynamic efficiency if, instead of having a single medium-sized vein, they have two smaller veins accompany the artery. These veins are referred to as venae comitantes. On seeing these small, shriveled-up structures in the dissecting room cadaver and learning the diminutive name applied to them, students gain an incorrect impression of the size and complexity of the veins and their interrelationships as they accompany the arteries. Likewise, their postmortem appearance gives no indication of the carrying capacity, potential size, and fragility of some of these vessels. The major axial veins have already been described in conjunction with the regional description of the arteries.

The second component of the deep system of veins of the lower extremity are the muscle sinuses. These are thin-walled intramuscular venous collecting systems. They are highly specialized capacitance vessels that empty into the venous drainage of the highly metabolically active muscle of the calf and, to a lessor extent, into the thigh. The structures run longitudinally in the muscle bellies. After leaving the muscle belly, in particular the gastrocnemius and soleus muscles, the veins turn forward to enter the posterior tibial and peroneal veins before coalescencing into the popliteal vein. These highly specialized systems allow the collection of large volumes of blood during times of peak exercise, and they are a mechanism of returning venous blood with increased energy into the axial venous system.

The third component of the deep venous system are the perforating or communicating veins. The perforators collect blood from many small veins ramifying in the subcutaneous tissue and the skin along with elements of the long saphenous vein. Thus, skin and subcutaneous tissue of the lower leg have a dual venous drainage system. Those venules that eventually coalesce into the perforating veins enter a short, thick, stubby vein that perforates the deep fascia and enters into the main axial veins.

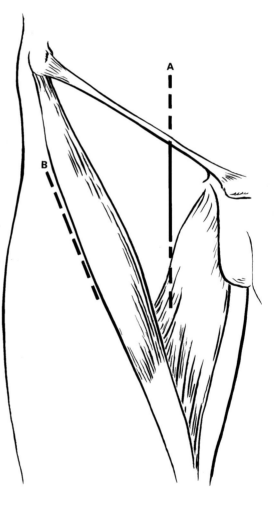

Figure 9-6. Illustration of the proximal thigh depicting a vertical incision A (*dotted and solid lines*) and oblique incision B (*dotted lines*). A is used in femoral bifurcation exposures. B is used in distala exposure of profunda femoris artery.

There are no short thick veins draining from the long saphenous vein into the deep veins of the calf or thigh. There are, however, direct communications between some of the muscular veins and the main axial veins and a more posteriorly placed arch of superficial veins called the posterior arch vein. The perforators are found approximately 5, 10 to 12, and about 20 cm or so above the medial malleolus. On the lateral aspect of the leg, there are frequently two perforators found at a variable distance above the lateral malleolus. There is usually one perforator in the thigh.

Superficial Veins

The superficial veins of the lower extremity include the long saphenous vein and its tributaries and the short saphenous vein and its tributaries.

Long Saphenous Vein

The long saphenous vein begins as a continuation of the superficial venous arch of the foot in front of the lateral malleolus. From there it passes superiorly and posteriorly to go behind the midpoint of the leg at the level of the knee joint. It then sweeps upward in a gentle curve on the inner aspect of the thigh to finally pierce the deep fascia in the femoral triangle through the fossa ovalis and thus gain entry into the common femoral vein.

At the saphenous opening just before perforating the deep fascia, it is joined by four or five major tributaries called the superficial circumflex iliac vein, superficial epigastric vein, the external pudendal vein, medial accessory saphenous vein, and lateral accessory saphenous vein. These terminations are extremely variable, and it is only by careful dissection in any individual subject that the true number of communications at the level of the fossa ovalis can be determined. The saphenous opening lies immediately behind the groin crease and medial to the pulse of the common femoral artery.

Short Saphenous Vein

The short saphenous vein begins as a continuation of the lateral marginal vein of the foot behind the medial malleolus. Initially it ascends on the lateral border of the Achilles tendon before achieving the midline of the back of the leg, where it ascends toward the popliteal space. Although classically described as perforating the deep fascia between the heads of the gastrocnemius in the lower part of the popliteal fossa and entering the popliteal vein above the level of the knee joint, the short saphenous vein has a much more variable relationship to the knee crease and entry into the popliteal vein than that description implies. The anatomy of the superficial veins of the lower extremity can be well mapped with duplex scanning.

EXPOSURES OF THE VESSELS OF THE LOWER EXTREMITY

The patient should be positioned supine. The legs should be well supported, and the heels positioned so that they are about 30 cm apart. The feet are allowed to rotate externally naturally.

A vertical or slightly curvy linear skin incision is made directly over the common femoral artery (Fig. 9-6). This incision crosses the groin crease for all groin exposures but will have different lengths above and below the crease depending on the pathology to be overcome and the purpose of the proposed procedure. For most aortofemoral grafting procedures to a relatively undiseased femoral system, the skin crease represents the middle of the wound. For femoropopliteal and profunda reconstructions, the length below the groin crease will be considerably greater than that above.

When a pulse is present at the common femoral artery, the incision is placed accordingly. When a pulse is absent, the incision should pass through a point on the inguinal ligament that is midway between the anterior superior iliac spine and the pubic symphysis, the so-called midinguinal point. This incision is made with a sharp scalpel, and the skin is divided cleanly, ensuring that the blade is held at right angles to the skin throughout the length of the cut. The skin is held at the appropriate tension by the surgeon and first assistant during the performance of the initial incision.

The wound may be developed further by sharp dissection using a scalpel to divide through the superficial fascia, avoiding the lymph nodes (Fig. 9-7). Any lymphatic trunks should be sealed by diathermy to prevent lymph leaks (Fig. 9-8). The only superficial structures apart from the lymph nodes and vessels are one or two superficial veins coursing from lateral to medial to join the long saphenous vein in the fossa ovalis, which cross in front of the common femoral artery. These veins should be ligated. This dissection proceeds with a clean incision to expose the femoral sheath, the inguinal ligament, and the lower fibers of external oblique muscle (Fig. 9-9).

An alternative methodology is to use a diathermy with blended cutting and coagulating currents. The skin edges are elevated and separated by hand-held rake-type retractors, and the diathermy needle is used to divide the tissue. The surgeon and assistant each hold a retractor and apply the required traction and countertraction to the skin edges to present the tissue for division. This method facilitates avoidance of the major lymph nodes and produces a dry wound. The superficial venous tributaries are dealt with by ligation.

Once the anterior lamella of the femoral sheath over the common femoral artery is on display, standard scissors and forceps dissection proceeds after the appropriate skin edge retraction and soft tissue retention have been established (Fig. 9-10).

We favor self-retaining retractor systems because they provide improved and stable visualization over hand-held retractors. Various types of retractor systems are applic-

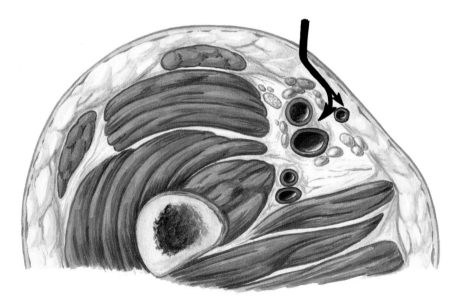

Figure 9-7. Cross-sectional view of the upper thigh. *Arrows* show the skin incision and the route to the vessel to expose the artery and relationships to the femoral and saphenous veins.

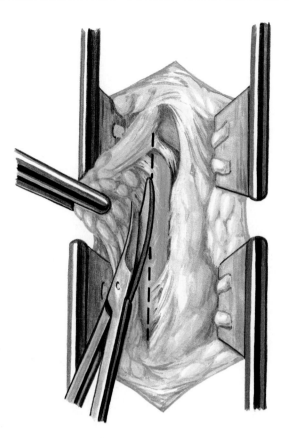

Figure 9-8. Deeper exposure with retraction and separation of lymphatics and exposure of fascia. The *dotted line* indicates the proposed incision in the femoral sheath.

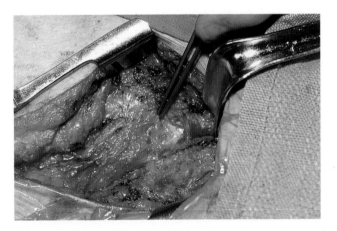

Figure 9-9. Operative photograph showing superficial exposure and retraction in the groin.

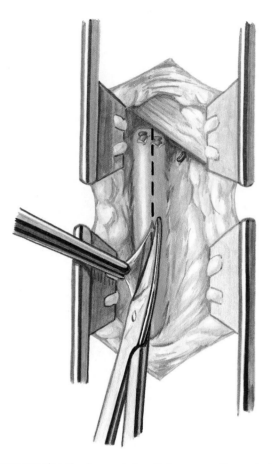

Figure 9-10. Surgeon opening the femoral sheath to expose the underlying femoral artery. The *dotted line* indicates the direction of the incision in the femoral sheath.

able. We tend to use the wishbone-mounted system, which is eminently suitable and enables all the required maneuvers in any groin operation to be accomplished. When wishbone systems are not available, the older spreading ratchet-type retractors are still suitable. We tend to use two retractors for each groin wound. The retractor lying along the thigh has straight handles, whereas the retractor inserted in the upper part of the wound has a handle with hinges in the middle of its length to enable conformity to the abdominal contours. These retractors lie well in the wound, and the use of two retractors spreads the tension of the skin and subcutaneous tissue more evenly while producing significantly better visualization, as the wound adopts a more rectangular profile rather than the diamond shape achieved by single self-retaining device. A hand-held retractor of the Langenbeck type is useful in elevating the inguinal ligament when the external circumflex iliac vein is ligated and divided.

Exposure of the Common Femoral Artery and Its Branches

Earlier in the chapter we described the initial skin incision and development of the superficial route to the front of the femoral sheath. When the roof of the femoral sheath over the artery is incised, the only structures at risk for damage are the femoral branch of the genitofemoral nerve and the branches of the femoral artery itself. The femoral vein and the branches of the femoral nerve are sequestered away in the other compartments of the femoral sheath and, even after circumferential mobilization of the artery, will be protected. This incision of the femoral sheath can easily be carried up to the inguinal ligament (Fig. 9-11).

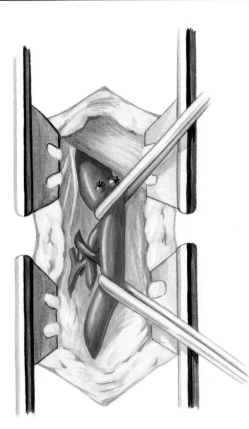

Figure 9-11. Exposure of profunda femoris artery with the circumflex femoral vein overlying the proximal profunda artery.

Once the inguinal ligament is on display, if an aortofemoral graft is to be placed, the lower edge of the inguinal ligament is elevated or divided (Fig. 9-12), and the anterior surface of the femoral artery is separated from it by retraction and elevation. The circumflex iliac vein is found coursing across in front of the terminal part of the external iliac artery (Fig. 9-13). This can be controlled with long straight clamps, and the vessel divided and ligated. This dissection is the beginnings of the retroperitoneal tunnel

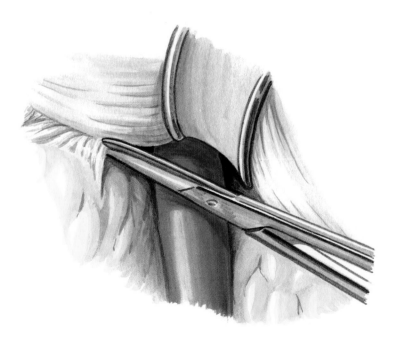

Figure 9-12. Lateral mobilization of inguinal region to facilitate elevating the inguinal ligament for proximal exposure of the external iliac–common femoral artery junction.

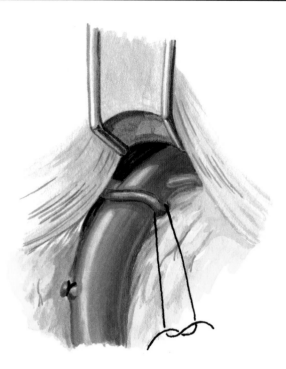

Figure 9-13. Circumflex iliac vein (vein of sorrow) crossing the distal external iliac artery above the level of the inguinal ligament.

from the groin exposure. Once the vein has been safety mobilized and suture ligated, the tunnel is easily developed on the lateral aspect of the external iliac artery, where it abuts on the iliac fascia covering the psoas major muscle. This component of the tunnel is made most easily in this area and also represents the safest anatomic route, as it avoids a substantial amount of the lymphatics. Careful attention to detail, with the finger being at all times in contact with the outer surface of the iliac artery, ensures that penetration of the peritoneum does not occur.

Inferiorly, the superficial femoral artery can be mobilized by distal continuation of the incision of the femoral sheath and the periadventitial tissue. The first 5 cm of

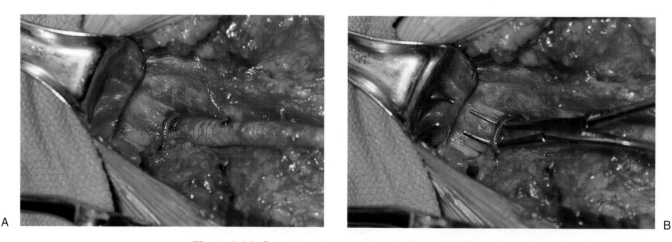

Figure 9-14. Operative photographs. **A:** Circumflex iliac vein crossing the distal external iliac artery. **B:** Clamp beneath the vein, opened in preparation for clamping and ligating the structure.

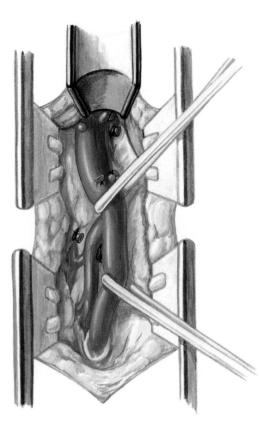

Figure 9-15. Soft plasma tubing slings used to elevate and displace the common femoral bifurcation to visualize the profunda origin. The lateral circumflex iliac vein branches have been divided to further visualize the proximal clip under femoris artery.

superficial femoral artery can easily be dissected and mobilized circumferentially (Fig. 9-14). Once the artery has disappeared behind the sartorius muscle, sharp dissection of the medial border of the sartorius muscle and lateral retraction of the muscle belly unroof the subsartorial canal. The superficial femoral artery can be dissected further distally.

This mobilization of the superficial femoral artery is also required to facilitate exposure of the profunda femoris vessel (Fig. 9-15). Once a length of superficial femoral artery has been exposed and mobilized, the origin of the profunda femoris is identified at the bifurcation. The origin of the profunda artery is dissected free of its investing periadventitial tissue. The first structure that dissection encounters is the circumflex femoral vein. This vein must be suture ligated and divided to permit access to the anterior surface of the profunda femoris artery. Once that has been done, the profunda trunk can be exposed to its distal third, where it pierces adductor magnus, by mobilization of the lateral margin of adductor longus muscle and the medial retention of that muscle belly. The lateral margin of adductor longus is dissected free and retracted medially to expose the continuing trunk of the profunda femoris artery. The caudal continuation of the groin dissection into the thigh is facilitated by mobilization and retention of the muscle bellies that cover and protect these important arteries as they course through the musculature of the thigh.

During femoropopliteal or femorodistal reconstructions, a tunnel must be formed from the femoral triangle and carried more distally into the leg. Three options are available: subcutaneous, subfascial, or a more anatomic placement of the tunnel to house the graft in the subsartorial canal. We regard anatomic placement of the tunnel as the best option. It is the safest and conforms best to our definition of exposure. It is also the most technically difficult to create in some patients, not in its upper extent but in the area of adductor hiatus. However, these potential technical difficulties are far outweighed by the advantages of following the natural pathway, with viable muscle tissue surrounding the graft and good control of fluid and blood accumulations as a result of the absence of dead space.

To begin the subsartorial tunnel from the groin exposure, the apex of the femoral triangle is widened, and a finger is inserted on the anterolateral aspect of the superficial femoral artery. The dissecting finger is advanced, with the fingernail kept in contact with the arterial wall. If required, a rigid tunneling device can be used to broaden the tunnel. Maintenance of the position behind sartorius, below the quite strong musculofascial roof of the canal, and anterolateral to the artery avoids any potential injury to nervous or venous structures within the canal. Damage to the saphenous nerve within the canal is a source of some morbidity to patients, and careful attention to the tunneling avoids that problem.

If required, the tunnel can be created subfascially by beginning underneath the fascia lata, extending across the sartorius into the groove between sartorius and gracilis, and entering the popliteal space between sartorius and gracilis. This offers the best and lowest-risk route of the tunnel in the subfascial space. Although some surgeons prefer to place the tunnel using the subcutaneous space, and particularly the site of harvest of the long saphenous vein, this is our least preferred option (Fig. 9-16).

At the completion of the mobilization, it has become our practice to review critically the wound and its components, including the routes to the artery and any tunnels so formed. We do this before performing the index operation and before heparin has been given. At that time, any areas of bleeding or any injury to lymph nodes that had previously been unrecognized are attended to with excision of the node, diathermy of small bleeding points, and ligature of any obvious vascular or lymphatic channels. We believe that at the completion of the vascular exposure, if the index procedure in that anatomic area is not to proceed immediately, the retraction and retention should be released to prevent unnecessary pressure on the wounds when complete retraction and retention are not required for access.

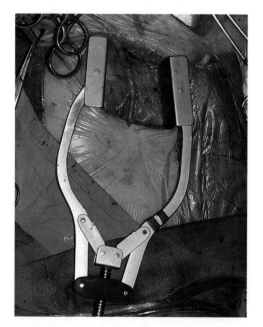

Figure 9-16. Operative photograph of groin exposure held by mechanical retractor. Note the mobilized external iliac artery above and the proximal superficial femoral artery below.

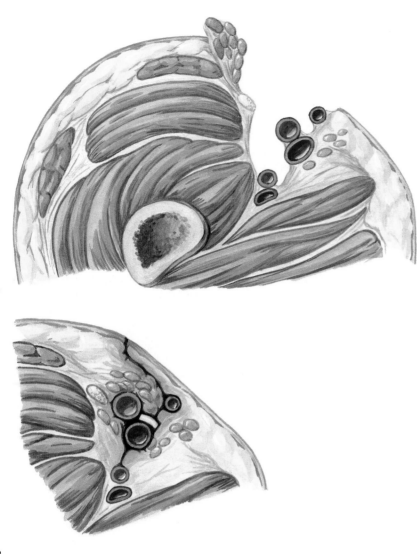

Figure 9-17. Steps in restoration of a groin incision. **A:** Cross section before wound closure. **B:** Placement of a drain adjacent to the vessels and a layered approximation of the wound to eliminate dead space.

Restoration

The restoration of the groin wound is consequent on the wound engineering that has gone into creating the exposure (Fig. 9-17). Adherence to the hierarchy of healing priorities, in any operative vascular intervention, is required to provide the optimum environment for the vascular wound to heal. The vascular wound itself requires coverage with viable tissue; thus, the perivascular structures must be coapted. The route of access to the vessel and the skin must be returned to as near normal as possible. In the previously unoperated groin, the tissue planes that hold suture material well include the femoral sheath, the fascia lata, the membranous layer of the superficial fascia, and the immediate subcuticular tissue. Thus, it is possible to coapt without tension four layers in most patients having their groin opened.

Although classical teaching has been that the femoral sheath should not be closed over implanted grafts because of a concern about compression, it has become our practice to do so. Femoral sheath is a resilient structure. It holds sutures well and is capable of bringing healthy, well-vascularized tissue in direct contact with the arterial wound. Coaptation of the sheath excludes the layers of fatty and lymphatic-rich tissue above, which are potential sources of contaminated or sterile fluid accumulation. Thus, we attempt to ensure a tension-free closure of the femoral sheath in all cases of primary arterial repair and in all cases where it is technically possible when a graft is in position. This can be accomplished as a separate layer. Frequently we use a somewhat different technique. A suture can begin at the level of the inguinal ligament and, sewing inferiorly, close the femoral sheath. The suture is brought back in the layer of the fascia lata, providing a secure fascial closure totally excluding the superficial lymph nodes from any capacity to leak onto the arterial repair. When the membranous layer of superficial fascia is closed, careful attention to detail of the alignment of the skin wound should be given during the closure. Appropriate corrective action should be taken by taking slightly bigger bites on one side or the other during the closure of that layer to ensure that the skin is aligned and evenly spaced on both sides of the wound. If the membranous layer of superficial fascia is closed carefully, a very fine subcuticular layer ensures tension-free coaptation of the skin. Thus, the principles we try to embody are a firm closure over the arterial wound and repair, coaptation of the routes of access, and tension-free approximation of the skin.

As stated earlier, if lymph nodes are damaged during the exposure, these are excised. If there is accumulation of fluid consistently in the wound with no obvious source, a drain is placed to the layers between the fascia lata and membranous layer of the superficial fascia to ensure obliteration of dead space and removal of any accumulated fluid. The drains are brought out through a separate stab incision, conforming to our practice and beliefs of exposure with separate exit wound and particular route of access to achieve the specific purpose of the suction drain.

The Reoperative Groin

A common phenomenon for us has been the necessity to reoperate in a groin that has been previously opened either to repair some complication of a previously placed aortofemoral or femoropopliteal graft or to originate a more distally seeking graft after a proximal reconstruction.

Depending on the pathology, the reoperative groin may be technically challenging, but on most occasions the reexploration is tedious. Our experience has led us to believe that the most important principle to be adopted is to try and convert the scarred previous operative field to as near "primary operative condition by the end of the procedure as is possible." This implies the redevelopment of the access route that the original surgeon took to the vessel, the identification and mobilization of the vessels, and, when it is safe to do so, the excision of as much of the previously laid-down scar tissue as is practical before closure restoration. It is surprising how narrow the fibrous scarred zone is in groins that have been previously operated on diligently, left dry, and in which there were no healing complications. Groins where there was previous superficial infection or lymphocoeles frequently have widely dispersed areas of scar and anomalous healing, which make the goal of attainment of normal restoration more difficult.

The patient is positioned similarly to the position used in the primary operation, the original skin scar is incised (Fig. 9-18), and the scar tissue is followed so that the original surgeon's steps are faithfully retraced (Fig. 9-19). In the dense scar of the reoperative wound, we sometimes use sharp-pointed tenotomy scissors to establish and continue appropriate paths to the vessels. In addition, the fine handles and small cutting area of the blades allow successful performance of periarterial dissection of previously mobilized arteries with minimal risk of arterial injury.

Once the level of the reconstituted femoral sheath has been attained, it is frequently easier to dissect more proximally and mobilize and trace a previous aortofemoral graft to the femoral artery. Alternatively, it may be desirable to proceed more distally, find previously undissected vessels, and mobilize these circumferentially. The aims of both maneuvers is the same: to ensure that the vascular mobilization is carried out in the

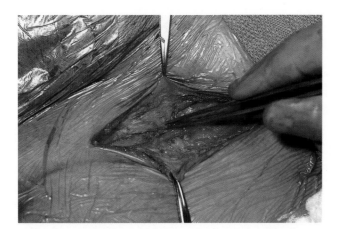

Figure 9-18. Operative photograph of the beginning of a reoperative groin exposure.

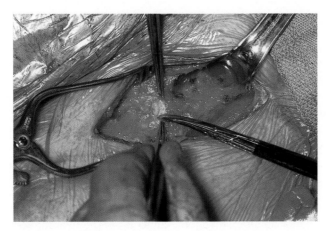

Figure 9-19. Operative photograph of a deeper dissection through scar tissue of a reoperative groin exposure.

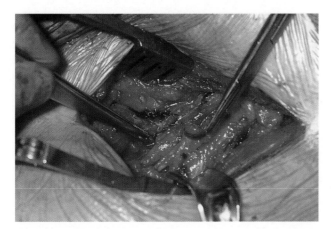

Figure 9-20. Operative photograph of the beginning dissection of the femoral vessels in the reoperative groin exposure.

true periadventitial plane (Fig. 9-20), thereby minimizing the risks to the artery itself and the surrounding structures.

Vessels that are patent even though they have been mobilized previously attempt to regenerate the plane of Leriche, and it is easier to identify this reformed plane if a previously undissected adjacent artery is mobilized and the depth for the proper dissec-

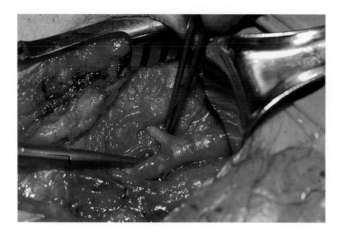

Figure 9-21. Operative photograph of the final mobilization of femoral artery and its bifurcation in a reoperative groin.

tion plane is established. A previously implanted graft, once it has been mobilized from its perigraft capsule, will also lead the surgeon to the correct dissection plane.

Thus, in general, the plan for the previously operated groin is to carefully retrace the original surgeon's footsteps, because a preestablished route of access has already been shown to be safe. Then it is possible to establish the appropriate level of dissection and then to remobilize the arteries circumferentially as required (Fig. 9-21). The appropriate excision of scar tissue and replacement of this with well-vascularized normal tissue is our goal before and during restoration, which should follow the previously described pattern. Suction drainage is mandatory.

Lateral Approach to the Branches of the Femoral Artery

On occasion, pathology in the groin, such as infection within the femoral triangle, precludes or demands an alternative route of access to the femoral vessels. Again, the anatomy of the region is brought into play (Fig. 9-22).

The incision is made beginning 2 to 3 inches below the anterior superior iliac spine and along the lateral margin of the sartorius. This incision is deepened, the lateral margin of sartorius is elevated, and a clean dissection plane behind sartorius is used to identify the superficial femoral and profunda femoris arteries (Fig. 9-23). In this exposure, the muscle belly of sartorius is retained medially, and if required, the medial side of adductor longus is mobilized and retained laterally to expose the mid third of the profunda femoris artery (Fig. 9-24).

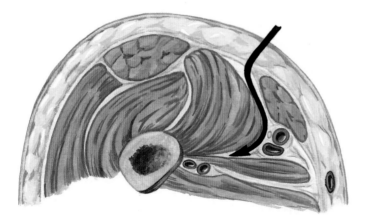

Figure 9-22. Cross section of the anterolateral approach to the groin. Note the course of the incision around the vastus medialis muscle to expose the profunda femoris artery. Site at the *arrow.*

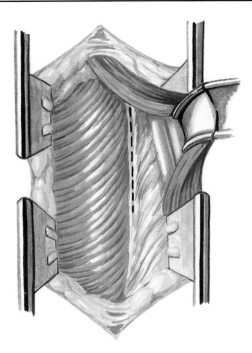

Figure 9-23. Anterolateral superficial exposure in the proximal thigh. The *dotted line* depicts the site of the fascial incision to expose the profunda femoris artery.

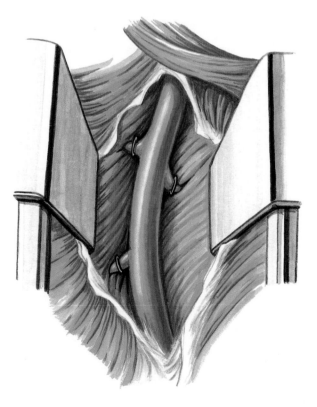

Figure 9-24. Mid- and distal trunk of the profunda femoris artery through anterolateral approach.

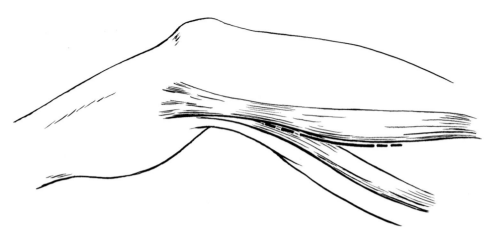

Figure 9-25. Incision for exposure of the superficial femoral artery in the midthigh (*dotted line*).

Thus, the femoral vessels can be approached through clean tissue planes to provide suitable access for an extraanatomic bypass in a clean exposure, excluding an area of contamination or frank sepsis. Conceptually, this accords with our principles of exposure and allows for precise restoration of anatomy at the completion of the vascular procedure.

Exposure of the Superficial Femoral Artery

The proximal superficial femoral artery is best exposed through the vertical groin incision described above. If required, an extension of the skin incision can be made distally. With appropriate lateral retraction of the sartorius, the proximal 10 to 15 cm of the superficial femoral artery is able to be exposed.

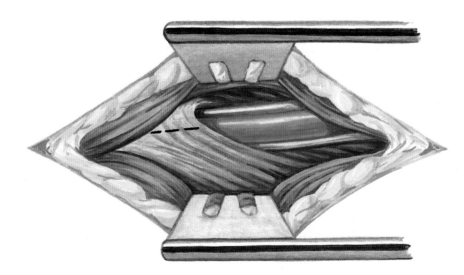

Figure 9-26. Deepened dissection and retraction showing exposed distal superficial femoral artery to the level of Hunter's canal. The *dotted line* shows the proposed incision to divide the adductor tendon.

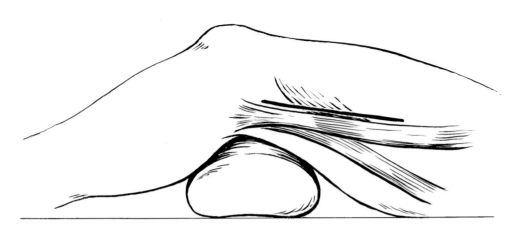

Figure 9-27. Medial supragenicular incision for exposure of the popliteal artery.

The whole of the remainder of the superficial artery can be exposed by an incision placed on the medial side of the thigh at the posterior border of sartorius (Fig. 9-25). In the lower thigh, this brings the dissection into the groove between sartorius anteriorly and gracilis posteriorly. Slightly higher in the thigh, the incision must be carried more anteriorly to follow the sweep of the sartorius muscle. An incision of appropriate length is made and deepened through the subcutaneous fat. The deep fascia of the leg is incised in the line of the wound and opened longitudinally for the length of the wound. The posterior border of sartorius is identified and cleaned. The muscle is then retracted anteriorly, and the canal is entered. A self-retaining retractor system is used to retain the soft tissue out of the field, and the superficial femoral artery can be mobilized circumferentially as far as is required. The only major structure at risk in this exposure is the long saphenous vein. If the wound has been correctly placed, this structure will usually be found in the posterior flap, slightly behind the margin of the incision (Fig. 9-26).

Restoration

This wound does not create dead space, so unless oozing is a problem, no drains are required. Closure of the deep fascia approximates all the deep tissues. This is accomplished with a running suture of absorbable material. The superficial fascia is closed in its membranosus layer, and the skin is approximated.

Exposure of the Popliteal Artery

Suprageniculate Popliteal Artery

The patient is positioned supine, and the leg to be operated on is prepared and draped free in the sterile field. The knee is flexed, and the lower extremity is allowed to rotate externally. The knee is supported on a drape-wrapped bowl or an unwrapped gown bundle. The incision begins at the medial condyle of the femur and is carried proximally in the long axis of the limb in the groove between sartorius and gracilis muscles (Fig. 9-27). The incision is deepened, and the deep fascia is divided in the line of the wound. The posterior border of sartorius is cleaned and retracted anteriorly. For exposure of the suprageniculate popliteal with the knee flexed, usually none of the muscles are required to be divided. However, on occasion the medial head of the gas-

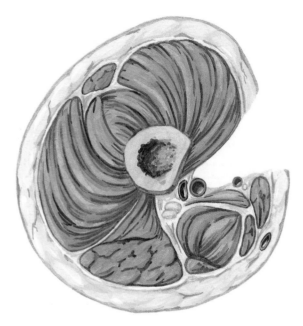

Figure 9-28. Cross section showing incision to expose the proximal popliteal artery and vein.

trocnemius can be an impediment and so should be incised to obtain the exposure necessary (Fig. 9-28). The artery is identified in the fat of the popliteal space and can be readily dissected by forceps and scissors dissection. There are usually two or three crossing veins that require ligation and division to fully expose the suprageniculate popliteal artery (Fig. 9-29). Performing this incision with the knee flexed allows access to the popliteal artery from its entry into the popliteal space to its intercondylar segment without muscular division.

The structures at risk during this mobilization include the long saphenous vein and, on occasion, the saphenous nerve. The major axial nerves are still remote from the artery at this level.

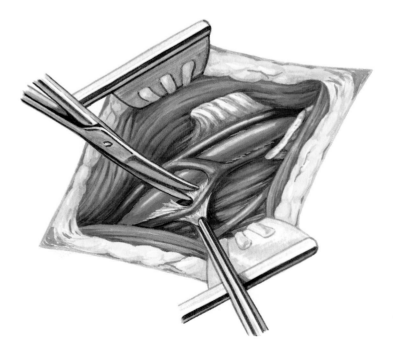

Figure 9-29. Exposure of the popliteal artery after division of the adductor tendon. Ligation of plexus periarterial venous is shown.

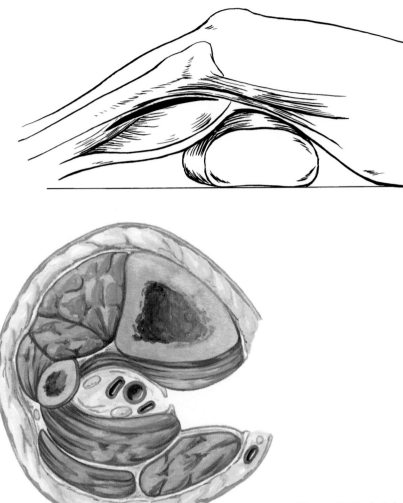

A

B

Figure 9-30. A: Infrapopliteal and medial exposure of the popliteal artery. **B:** Cross-sectional view of this exposure.

Restoration

Entry into the popliteal fossa always creates dead space. There is no mechanism to obliterate the dead space using tissue approximation, so that some free fluid formation in the space is inevitable. If we adopt the principles espoused in **Chapter 1** and illustrated in **Chapter 2**, it would then follow that all wounds of the popliteal space should be drained. Drainage is required for only a short period of time, and a fine multiholed closed suction drainage system prevents fluid accumulation and ensures coverage of the artery by healthy viable tissue. The suction drain should be brought out through a separate stab incision. Closure is effected by approximating the deep fascia using a continuous suture. Coaptation of the membranosus layer of the superficial fascia and approximation of the skin completes the restoration.

Exposure of the Infrageniculate Popliteal Artery

The infrageniculate popliteal artery is exposed through a medial incision placed posterior to the bony prominence of the tibia. It extends from the tibial tuberosity distally for about 10 cm (Fig. 9-30). The subcutaneous tissue and the deep fascia are

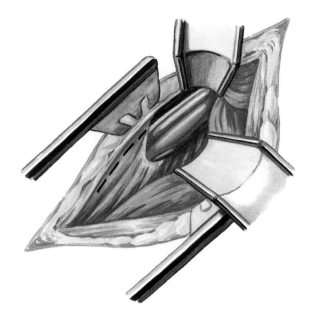

Figure 9-31. Illustration of the popliteal artery and vein. The *dotted line* shows the line of division of the soleus from the tibia to extend the arterial exposure distally.

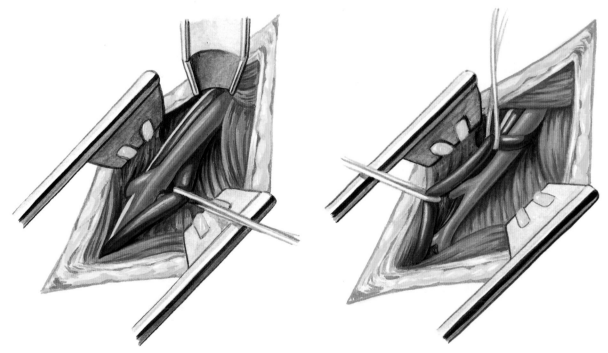

A

B

Figure 9-32. A: Illustration of the exposed terminal popliteal artery and the anterior tibial origin. The posterior tibial nerve is deep. **B:** The popliteal vein is elevated with slings.

incised in the line of the wound. In the base of the wound, the medial head of the gastrocnemius is identified, and the anterior border is cleaned. This muscle is retracted posteriorly, and access to the space is obtained. The artery can be felt in the floor of the fossa anterior to the nerve trunks and, at this stage of its course, partly obscured on the medial side by the popliteal vein.

Although this is the classical description of the infrageniculate approach, usually the incision has to be carried more proximally and distally to expose the midpopliteal artery and, in patients with extensive atherosclerosis, the tibioperoneal trunk and anterior tibial arteries. The proximal extension of this infrageniculate incision carries the skin incision along the line described for the suprageniculate approach. After the deep fascia is divided, the tendons of gracilis, semimembranosus, and semitendinosus are divided along the line of the wound, and the medial head of the gastrocnemius can be divided from its origin on the femoral condyle. Division of these muscles allows the exposure of the whole of the popliteal artery from its beginning in the adductor hiatus to the termination as it passes behind the arch of soleus (Fig. 9-31). Division of the arch of soleus and longitudinal extension along the line of the posterior tibial artery allow the dissection of the primary branches of the tibioperoneal trunk for the requisite distance to perform any index operation in that region (Fig. 9-32).

The distal popliteal and tibioperoneal trunk have a well-developed and thin-walled venous network that surrounds them. The venae comitantes of the anterior tibial, posterior tibial, and peroneal arteries are also adherent to those structures, and there are numerous crossing veins joining the venae comitantes. When atherosclerosis is present in these vessels, the inflammatory component of that disease causes even tighter adherence of these periarterial structures, and troublesome bleeding can occur if great care is not used in the dissection.

In addition to the periarterial venous network and venae comitantes, the major axial nerves have reached a closer relationship with the artery in the infrageniculate popliteal fossa and are closely approximated as the vessels pass beneath the tendinous origin of soleus muscle. Therefore, these structures are at risk for damage during this dissection. The saphenous vein, of course, remains at risk in the superficial part of the wound.

Restoration

Complete exposure of the infrageniculate segment or the whole of the popliteal artery creates dead space that is not able to be obliterated using the standard repair techniques. Thus, suction drainage is mandatory. Usually for the complete drainage of the popliteal space, two 3-mm suction catheters are laid to exit above and below the primary wound and remove the inevitable collection of extracellular fluid and lymph from the space, thus facilitating approximation of healthy tissue over the vascular wounds. The divided muscles are repaired using nonabsorbable suture material. The deep fascia is closed in a continuous layer using absorbable suture material, whereas the membranosus layer of the superficial fascia and the skin are approximated.

Posterior Exposure of the Popliteal Artery

On occasion, it may be easier to approach the popliteal artery from its posterior aspect. A vertical incision is placed over the roof of the popliteal fossa between the medial and lateral hamstring muscles, crossing the joint line and extending inferiorly between the two heads of the gastrocnemius muscle (Fig. 9-33). The structures immediately at risk during the creation of this incision include the short saphenous vein and the medial cutaneous nerve of the leg. When the heads of the gastrocnemius and the hamstrings are retracted and retained apart, the first structures seen are the main trunk and branches of the posterior tibial nerve. The common peroneal nerve is liable for damage during retention of the structures because it is closely related to the muscle and tendon of biceps femoris in the supralateral margin of the popliteal space. The tibial nerve should be mobilized. It is safest to develop a route of access to the vessels on

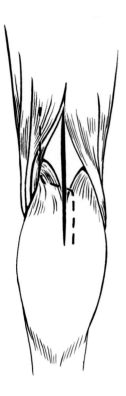
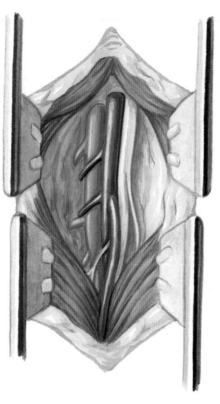

A,B

Figure 9-33. **A:** Preferred (*solid line*) and optional (*dotted line*) sites for skin incisions to expose the popliteal artery. **B:** The popliteal artery, vein, and posterior tibial nerve are visualized through this longitudinal posterior exposure.

the medial side of this axial nerve. The only nerve liable for damage on that side is the nerve to the medial head of the gastrocnemius. When the popliteal artery is the subject of aneurysm, the tibial nerve is displaced from its midline position and may be found on the lateral or medial side of the enlarged popliteal artery. When the tibial nerve has been satisfactorily mobilized and retracted laterally, the popliteal vessels are visualized, with the vein being a posteromedial relation of the artery through its course through the popliteal space. Thus, the vein must be dissected from the vessel before the artery can be circumferentially mobilized. Access can be gained through this incision to the whole of the length of the popliteal artery.

Restoration

Because this wound creates dead space, suction drainage is obligatory, and a standard closure of the deep fascia, subcutaneous tissue, and skin completes a satisfactory anatomic restoration.

Medial Approach to the Posterior Crural Arteries

In the lower one-third of the calf, the posterior tibial artery is a superficially placed vessel after it emerges from under cover of the soleus and gastrocnemius. In this part of the calf, it is covered only by skin, thin subcutaneous tissue, and investing deep fascia and lies approximately 2.5 cm anterior to the Achilles tendon. Thus, an incision placed directly over the artery behind flexor digitorum longus, deepened through the skin, and dividing the fascia will provide direct exposure of the posterior tibial artery (Fig. 9-34). The artery is of substantial size and good quality in this region and can be easily mobilized away from its venae comitantes and the accompanying posterior tibial nerve.

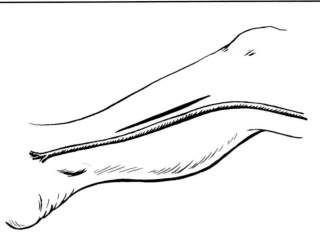

Figure 9-34. Proposed line of incision in the medial calf to expose the posterior tibial and peroneal artery.

Restoration of this wound requires no drains because no dead space is created and the deep fascia can be closed with simple approximation of the skin.

Throughout the calf it is possible to access the whole length of the posterior tibial artery via the medial approach. Similarly, it is through this approach that the peroneal artery can be accessed in the lower two-thirds of the calf. The incision is made behind the posterior border of the tibia and carried as far proximal and distal as required. The deep fascia is incised for the length of the wound (Fig. 9-35). An intermuscular plane is established between flexor digitorum longus anteriorly and the soleus–gastrocnemius group posteriorly. With attention to the establishment of this plane, retraction of the skin wound, and continuous adjustment of the retention of the soft tissues, the plane can be rapidly and easily established through loose areolar tissue to expose the posterior tibial neurovascular bundle. The venae comitantes of the artery is the first structure seen; then the artery and the lateral veins appear, with the posterior tibial

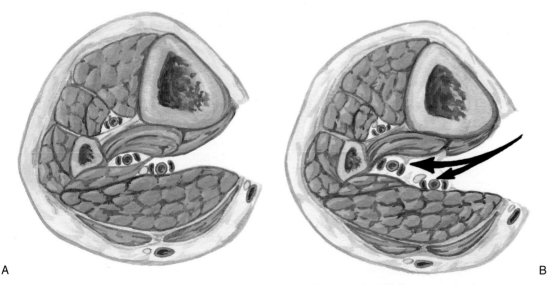

A   B

Figure 9-35. A: Cross-sectional view of the incision with the posterior tibial artery and vein exposed. **B:** Cross section of the approach extended more medially to visualize the peroneal artery and vein is shown. (*Arrows* identify the vascular structures.)

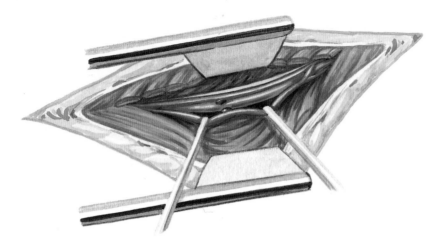

Figure 9-36. Medially placed longitudinal incision to expose the posterior tibial artery and nerve.

nerve occupying the lateral component of the posterior tibial neurovascular bundle. With an adequate length of skin incision and the proper retraction displacing soleus backward, adequate space can be created in front of that muscle for access to circumferential mobilization of and operative intervention on the posterior tibial vessel (Fig. 9-36). The structures at risk during this exposure include the long saphenous vein and saphenous nerve, the accompanying veins of the tibial artery as well as the artery itself, and, of course, the tibial nerve, which has a close relationship in the neurovascular bundle.

Peroneal Artery

The dissection we have already described to expose the posterior tibial artery can be extended behind the posterior tibial neurovascular bundle to develop a plane between tibialis posterior and the flexor hallucis longus muscle (Fig. 9-37). At the base of that intermuscular septum, the fibrous sheath surrounding the peroneal artery and its venae comitantes can be entered, with the first structure encountered being the medial vena comitantes of the artery. The key to this dissection is a meticulous following of the intermuscular septa. Posterior retraction of the soleus–gastrocnemius through an adequate skin incision with retention of the posterior tibial neurovascular bundle anteriorly facilitates the clear demarcation of the septum between the deeply placed tibialis posterior and the flexor hallucis longus.

Restoration

At the completion of the index procedure, closure of the deep fascia enables an anatomic restoration of the route to the vessels to be approximated. Thus, unless there is considerable oozing in the wound, drains are not required. The closure of the deep fascia of the leg accomplishes an anatomic restoration, leaving only the membranous layer of the superficial fascia and skin to be approximated.

Lateral Exposure of the Peroneal Artery

The peroneal artery can be exposed from the lateral side in the middle part of the calf by excising the middle third of the fibula. The incision is placed to overlay the intermuscular septum, which divides the peroneal compartment from the posterior muscular compartment and thus is in the groove between the gastrocnemius muscle and the peroneus longus. The subcutaneous tissue can be divided, and the deep fascia incised, to bring the surgeon to the fibula. The periosteum of the fibula is then incised, and a subperiosteal resection of the middle third of the fibula is performed. In the base of the wound, the periosteum of the medial side in front of flexor hallucis longus is divided. The wound and this dissection open the lateral aspect of the peroneal vascular bundle. Excision of the fibula, anterior retraction of the peroneal muscles, and posterior retraction of the soleus–gastrocnemius group facilitate this exposure, which allows circumferential mobilization of the peroneal artery for the whole of the extent of bony excision.

Restoration

The exposure should be drained routinely, as dead space and oozing are inevitable after resection of the fibula. A small suction drain is all that is required. It is not usually possible to close the deep fascia, so the only available cover for this wound would be superficial fascia and skin approximation.

Exposures of the Anterior Tibial Artery

Like the posterior tibial artery the anterior tibial artery is superficially placed in the lower one-third of the leg. It can be exposed in the distal third of the leg by a skin incision with division of the deep fascia parallel and medial to extensor hallucis longus. On the dorsum of the foot, the dorsalis pedis artery can be accessed through a skin and subcutaneous incision and division of the deep fascia lateral to the tendon of extensor hallucis longus, which crosses the vessel at the level of the ankle joint. These wounds are restored in the standard fashion.

Higher in the calf, the anterior tibial artery may be exposed by developing a route through the anterior compartment (Fig. 9-37). The anterior tibial artery is placed deep in the anterior compartment, lying in the front of the interosseous membrane. The best route of access to the vessel is through the intermuscular septum between tibialis anterior and extensor hallucis longus. This septum can usually be felt as a groove at the lateral border of the tibialis anterior muscle and allows direct access to the anterior tibial artery without violation of muscle bellies. An incision of sufficient length is made, the thin subcutaneous tissue is divided, and the deep fascia is incised in the line of the wound. The lateral border of the tibialis anterior is identified, and extensor hallucis longus, which lies somewhat more posterior, is identified subsequently. The intermus-

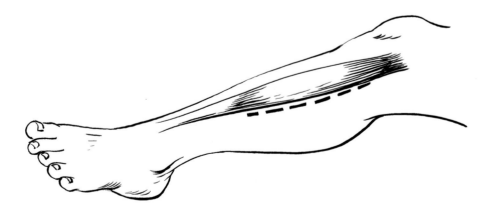

Figure 9-37. Proposed anterolateral incision (*dotted lines*) for exposure of the anterior tibial artery.

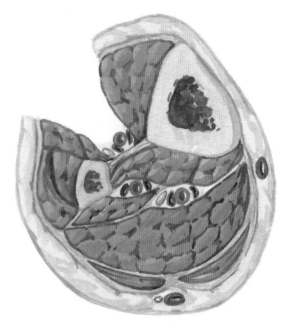

Figure 9-38. Cross-section of the proximal calf with the wound created to expose the route of entry to the artery and its accompanying vein and nerve.

cular septum is opened with careful incision (Fig. 9-38). No major structures are at risk until the neurovascular bundle is approached, when the venae comitantes and the deep peroneal nerve may be injured. The key to this exposure is adequate skin incision and lateral retraction of extensor hallucis longus as only slight medial retraction of the tibialis anterior is possible technically. In order to facilitate the exposure of the vessel, extensor hallucis longus must be mobilized all the way to the interosseous membrane. Once that has happened, and the muscle is retained, the vessels may be mobilized for the required distance (Fig. 9-39).

When the intermuscular dissection plane has been established, distal extension is possible as far as the dorsalis pedis, and the whole of the anterior tibial artery in the anterior compartment can be displayed.

On the medial side of the leg it is possible to display the whole of the vascular tree from the common femoral artery to the posterior tibial artery through a single incision

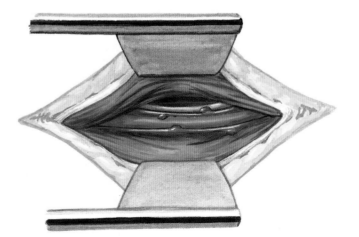

Figure 9-39. Longitudinal exposure of the anterior tibial artery and peroneal nerve in the anterolateral calf.

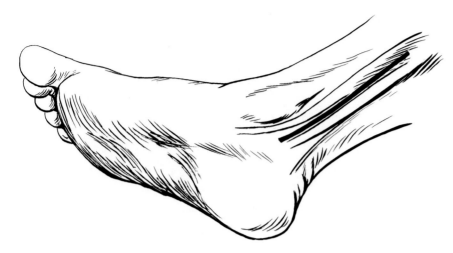

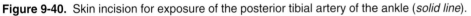

Figure 9-40. Skin incision for exposure of the posterior tibial artery of the ankle (*solid line*).

with division of only the structures around the knee joint, as described in the mobilization of the popliteal artery.

Anterior and Posterior Tibial Arteries at Ankle

The anatomy of these vessels, both of which are very superficially placed at the ankle, has been described. Both vessels are exposed by skin incision and division of superficial and investing fascia. The details are shown in Figs. 9-40 through 9-42. Restoration is usually accomplished by simple skin suture.

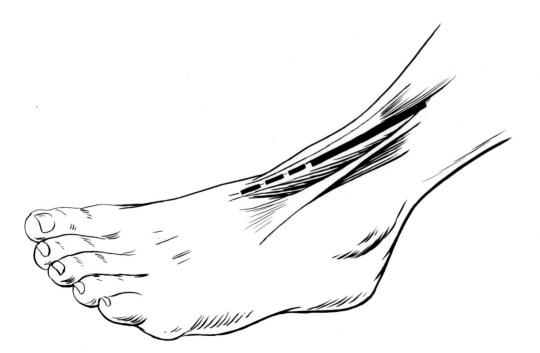

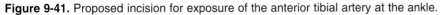

Figure 9-41. Proposed incision for exposure of the anterior tibial artery at the ankle.

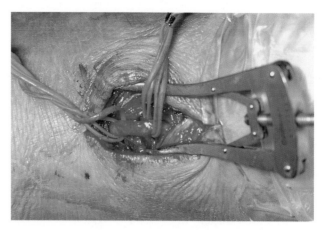

Figure 9-42. Operative photograph of the anterior tibial artery at the ankle.

Exposures of the Superficial Veins of the Lower Extremity

The superficial veins of the lower extremity are an important source of autogenous graft material for the vascular surgeon. With the ready availability of duplex scanning, there is now no reason to have doubts about the adequacy of the long saphenous vein or the short saphenous vein in any patient being considered for procedures requiring the use of these conduits. Duplex scanning allows an accurate mapping not only of the position of these venous structures but also of their size, whether they are double or bifid, etc. Thus, preoperative assessment may include indelible marking of the skin overlying the saphenous vein, precluding the need to ever have anything but direct incision over the vein if harvest of the vein is the only procedure being performed.

Harvest of the vein will still need to be performed through some incisions placed primarily to obtain access to the arteries. In these incisions, there is frequently the creation of some flaps with the potential for interference with blood supply and venous drainage of the flaps. These problems of wound engineering lead to fluid accumulation and other healing complications such as skin necrosis.

Termination of Long Saphenous Vein

The termination of the long saphenous vein can be exposed in the groin (Fig. 9-43). The incision is made in the groin crease medial to the femoral artery pulse and is extended for 3 to 4 cm. Scarpa's fascia is incised, and a small self-retaining retractor is used to spread the superficial tissue. If the incision has been placed correctly, the long saphenous vein is visible in the base of the wound. The long saphenous vein is grasped with the forceps and elevated while the dissection proceeds. It should be cleaned of its investing fascia to its junction with the common femoral vein, and this junction in the fossa ovalis should be demonstrated with certainty. There are usually four or five major tributaries that should be identified, cleaned, and divided. At the completion of the dissection of the saphenous vein in the fossa ovalis, there should be no doubt in the surgeon's mind that this is the termination of the saphenous vein and that there are no further tributaries entering it.

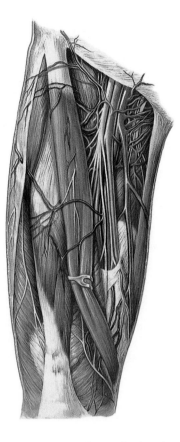

Figure 9-43. Saphenofemoral junction and related anatomy at the groin.

The Saphenous Vein at the Ankle

The saphenous vein can be usefully exposed at the ankle. The incision is placed on the anterior aspect of the ankle 2 cm anterior and superior to the medial malleolus. An incision of 2 to 3 cm is made. A curved artery forceps is used to spread the superficial tissue and the vein identified in the wound. It is elevated and freed for about 2 cm. Both of these wounds are restored by suture of the superficial fascia and approximation of the skin.

Similar closure is required for the harvest sites where the wounds are made longitudinally; however, in this case, if the vein is removed, there is the potential for dead space. Thus, it has become our practice to obliterate the site of venous procurement by continuous suture of the bed of the long saphenous vein or, if that is not possible, to drain the bed of the saphenous vein. The membranosus layer of the superficial fascia is then approximated over this closure, and the skin is approximated. Using this technique in combination with preoperative mapping of the saphenous vein has stopped some of the complications of saphenous vein harvest, including fluid collection and superficial infection.

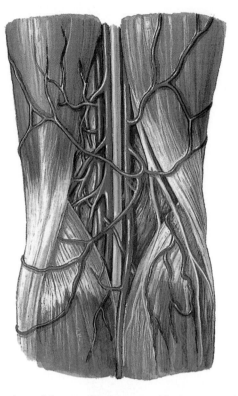

Figure 9-44. Posterior view of the popliteal space with the entry of the termination of the lesser saphenous vein at the end of the popliteal vein.

Termination of Short Saphenous Vein

The termination of the short saphenous vein should be located and mapped by ultrasound. The skin overlying it should be marked. The vein can then be exposed through a short skin-crease incision directly over the saphenopopliteal junction (Fig. 9-44). The skin incision can be deepened through the superficial fascia and fatty tissue of the popliteal space as required. Restoration is by simple suture approximation of the deeper structures and skin closure.

10
Tunnels

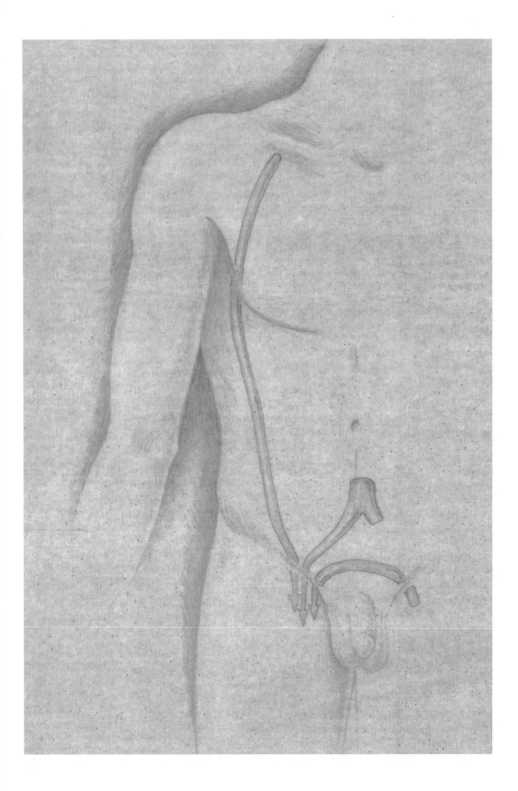

Tunnels are used frequently in vascular surgery. They are specialized wounds, usually designed to connect two sites of open vascular display. The wound we call a tunnel has been very much underestimated and is not often thought of as being part of exposure. Yet tunnels are often the source of morbidity, altered healing, and long-term problems for the patient.

Tunnels are created in various body spaces or potential spaces: subcutaneous, retroperitoneal, submuscular, or interfascial body compartments. They may be anatomic in the sense that they follow a path of a named neurovascular bundle, or extraanatomic, when the tunnel is remote from the arteries the conduit it contains will replace.

Tunnels are undoubtedly a wound and an important component of the concept of exposure, even though there may be no exposed artery or arterial wounds in their length. Tunnels may traverse a variety of structures, often more than one body region, and not infrequently they cross sites of active motion. Because of this, correct tunneling requires careful attention to the planning of procedures and precision in performance of the exposure and restoration as previously described. Atraumatic instrumentation along well-defined routes should be the norm. The routes chosen should avoid areas where predictable bleeding from arterial or venous damage or where leakage of lymph will be a problem. The concerns about tunnels are generally more significant in reoperative surgery, where the tunnel may be the most significant part of the procedure, requiring the engineering of a new wound in viable tissue, even though the scar of a previous incision and access route may have been reopened.

The tunnel created to allow the passage of a vascular graft is an unusual wound. Yet, as indicated above, the tunnel may be the source of considerable problems. During the conduct of the operation, there may be bleeding or injury to other tissues; in the immediate postoperative period, problems may arise in relation to collection of blood or tissue fluid. In the late postoperative period, if the tunnel had been constructed properly, healing and graft incorporation should be complete, but the patient may be left with residual seromata or, in the worst case, infection along the path of the graft.

The thesis we have developed throughout this volume is that the initial engineering of the wound determines in large part the fate of the artery, anastomosis, or graft that is surrounded by the healing environment. It has been our contention that the direct apposition of "normal tissue" over the artery so as to preclude dead space and fluid/blood accumulation is the optimal environment in which the arterial wound should heal. An extension of that logic to the vascular tunnel would lead to the thesis that tunnels should be as small as possible, consistent with the anatomic constraints related to placing the conduit. Tunnels should be dry, without blood or lymph leak at the time of graft placement, and if dead space cannot be obliterated by tissue apposition, then the tunnel should be drained by a closed suction drainage system.

THE AORTOFEMORAL TUNNEL

The exposures of the aorta and femoral arteries have been dealt with in **Chapters 2, 7, and 9.** The placement and the extent of the incisions required to expose these arteries have been described in detail. It is important to reiterate, however, that proximal dissection of the common femoral artery in the groin must always include the distal external iliac artery. To achieve this exposure, the lower fibers of the inguinal ligament are elevated or divided. The circumflex iliac vein is identified and divided where it crosses in front of the external iliac artery on its passage from lateral to medial to join the external iliac vein. Failure to undertake this step causes quite troublesome bleeding if the vein is injured during the construction of the retroperitoneal tunnel. Mobilization or division of the lower fibers of the inguinal ligament is a very important maneuver to provide access to the deeper structures, and the dissection allows the safe beginnings of the abdomen-to-groin tunnel for placement of the graft. This maneuver also prevents the complication of graft compression where the graft passes behind the inguinal ligament in its passage from the abdominal cavity to the groin.

The retroperitoneal tunnels required for aortofemoral bypass are best made by the use of the fingers. The index finger of one hand is placed from the retroperitoneal exposure of the right common iliac artery, while the index finger of the other hand is placed beneath the inguinal ligament. The fingernails are maintained on the anterolateral aspect of the external and common iliac arteries, and the fingers are advanced through the soft tissue in that periarterial plane until they meet. There are usually one or two areas of resistance felt along the path of this tunnel. A very important step in the creation of this tunnel is to ensure that the fingers pass behind the ureter to avoid compression of that structure after graft placement. The creation of the tunnel on the anterolateral aspect of the iliac artery represents not only the easiest anatomic path but also the safest anatomic route, as it avoids most of the lymphatics associated with the iliac artery system. Careful attention to the precision with which the finger is kept in contact with the outer surface of the iliac artery ensures that penetration of the peritoneum, with the attendant risk of visceral adhesion and fistula formation, does not occur and also that ureteric compression does not occur from the retroureteric path adopted by the graft. On the left-hand side, the periaortic component of the tunnel should be made behind the inferior mesenteric artery before following a path similar to that discussed for the right side.

Once the tunnel has been made, a long clamp can be passed over the inferior finger to meet the intraabdominal finger, which guides the clamp into the periaortic wound.

THE FEMORO-FEMORAL TUNNEL

On occasion it is necessary to cross from one femoral artery to the other to overcome unilateral iliac occlusion or, more commonly, to deal with graft sepsis. There are two possible routes for the femoro-femoral tunnel: subcutaneously or deep to the rectus abdominis through the space of Retzius.

The superficial tunnel is created by beginning a dissection in the upper aspect of the standard femoral wound, over the lower fibers of the external oblique aponeurosis. A satisfactory plane can be rapidly developed in front of the inguinal ligaments and external oblique aponeurosis on either side. Index fingers of both hands are then inserted into these openings and advanced toward each other, meeting in the midline above the pubis (Fig. 10-2). The tunnel is created deep behind the skin and subcutaneous tissue immediately in front of the external oblique aponeurosis. The tunnel created is usually bloodless, can be made rapidly, and avoids any risk of injury to the bladder that is sometimes associated with the creation of the tunnel through the space of Retzius.

On occasion, however, the more deeply placed tunnel is required. The tunnel is begun by elevation and mobilization of the inguinal ligament above the artery and the

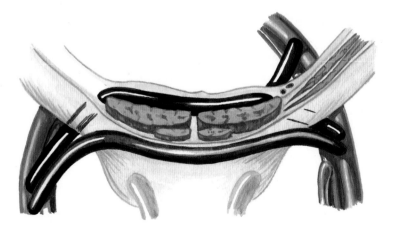

Figure 10-2. Femorofemoral tunnels.

division of the lower eighth of its fibers on both sides. A little sharp dissection in that plane allows the surgeon to place the index fingers of both hands behind the abdominal wall musculature, and keeping the fingers pressed against the posterior aspect of the anterior abdominal wall allows a path to be easily generated in the areolar tissue behind the lower fibers of rectus abdominis. The fingers meet easily, usually in the midline. The only structure at risk during the performance of this tunneling is the bladder, which is very unlikely to be injured if the tunnels are made with the fingers rather than a clamp or tunneling device. The same pathway can be used to route a graft from the iliac artery on one side to the femoral artery on the other.

THE AXILLOFEMORAL TUNNEL

Placement of an axillofemoral graft requires the creation of a long, initially submuscular and then subcutaneous, tunnel to link the axillary artery to the femoral artery. Exposure of the axillary artery has been described in **Chapter 8,** and the groin exposures have been discussed in **Chapters 2, 7, and 9.** Division of the pectoralis minor allows the formation of a funnel-like structure in the axillary wound. The index finger of the right hand can be placed into this beginning of the tunnel and passed

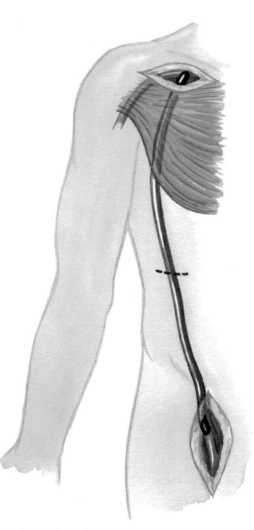

Figure 10-3. Axillofemoral tunnels, using a subclavicular and groin exposure. A third incision (*dotted line*) can be vased optionally.

down behind the fibers of pectoralis major in the anterior axillary line. In the groin, the tunnel is commenced anterior to the inguinal ligament, slightly to the lateral side of the common femoral artery, and sharp dissection is used to begin a deep subcutaneous tunnel. A long tunneling instrument is then passed from the groin, superficial to the chest wall musculature, eventually passing behind pectoralis major and up into the subclavicular wound to where it is guided by the operator's finger.

Although this maneuver can be accomplished, frequently a relieving incision is required over the lower chest wall in order to facilitate the correct alignment and satisfactory placement of the graft. This is always required if a short tunneler is the only instrument available (Fig. 10-3). Great care must be taken in making this incision through the skin and subcutaneous tissue to allow the tunneler to emerge and be reinserted without damage to the surrounding structures. It is important that the tunneler be kept against the muscles of the abdomen and the chest wall so that as much of the superficial tissue as is possible covers the graft. The alignment of the graft is also critical: it must be placed so as not to be kinked or compressed during the patient's sleep. In line with the principles outlined above, the tunneler should be as small as is compatible with anatomic placement of the graft.

UNUSUAL TRUNK TUNNELS

Ascending Aorta to Intraabdominal Aorta Bypass

Ascending aorta exposures through a median sternotomy have been developed in **Chapter 5**, and the abdominal aortic components are discussed in detail in **Chapter 7**. The graft is originated from the ascending aorta and is routed over the right atrium and along the right border of the heart but within the pericardium (Fig. 10-4). The exit point into the abdomen is a tunnel created in the pericardium and diaphragm in front of the aortic hiatus, and from there a tunnel can be developed in the retropancreatic plane to reach any part of the abdominal aorta. The combination of the supraceliac and infrarenal aortic exposures can be used, or, if required for a multiple vessel revascularization en route, a medial visceral rotation exposes the potential tunnel to its fullest extent.

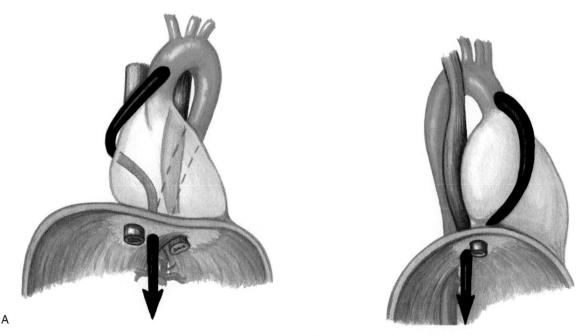

A   B

Figure 10-4. Ascending aorta to retroperitoneal tunnel: **(A)** anteroposterior and **(B)** lateral views.

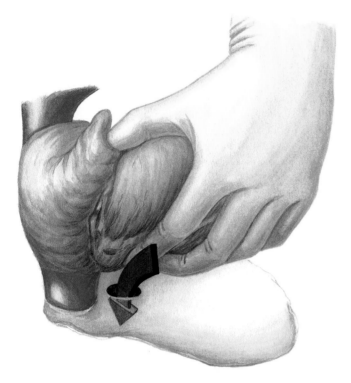

Figure 10-5. Upward retraction and left lateral rotation of the heart to visualize origin of tunnel in the inferior pericardial sac.

Descending Aorta to Iliac Artery Tunnel

Occasionally, because of difficulties in access to the infrarenal aorta, the descending thoracic aorta is the site of origin of the graft. The exposures of the thoracic aorta have been described in **Chapter 4**, and the visceral rotation components of the exposures in **Chapter 7**. The graft originates from the descending thoracic aorta, can be brought through the diaphragm (Fig. 10-5), and lies in the plane in front of the kidney to the left-hand side of the native aorta down to the iliacs, where it can be attached to one or other of those vessels (Fig. 10-6). The tunnel is reconstituted by tissue apposition over the graft that has been placed.

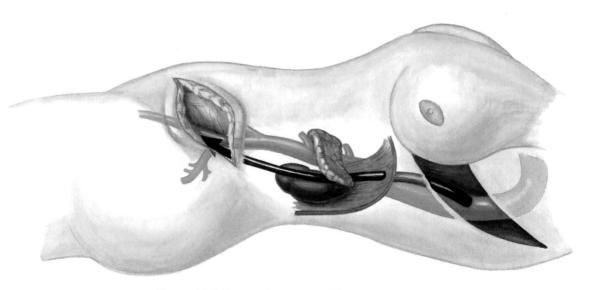

Figure 10-6. Descending aorta to iliac artery tunnel.

LEG TUNNELS

During femoro-popliteal or femoro-distal reconstructions, a tunnel is required to be formed from the femoral triangle and carried more distally into the leg. Three options are available: subcutaneous, subfascial, or a more anatomic placement of the tunnel to house the graft in a subsartorial canal. We regard the anatomic placement of the tunnel as the best option. It is the safest and conforms best to our definition of exposure. It is also the most technically difficult to create, not in its upper extent but mainly in the area of the adductor hiatus in some patients. However, the advantages of following the natural pathway include viable muscle tissue surrounding the graft and good control of fluid and blood accumulations, as there is no dead space; these far outweigh the potential technical difficulties.

To begin the subsartorial tunnel from the groin exposure, the apex of the femoral triangle is widened, and a finger is inserted onto the anterolateral aspect of the super-

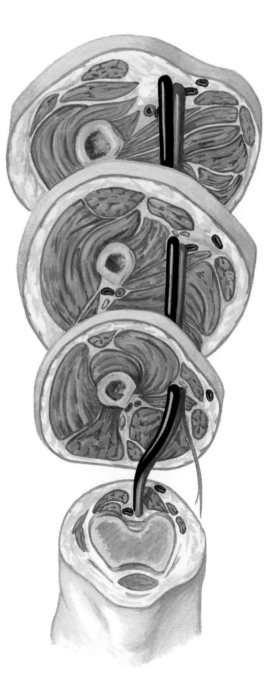

Figure 10-7. Subsartorial tunnel in cross-sectional anatomy of the thigh.

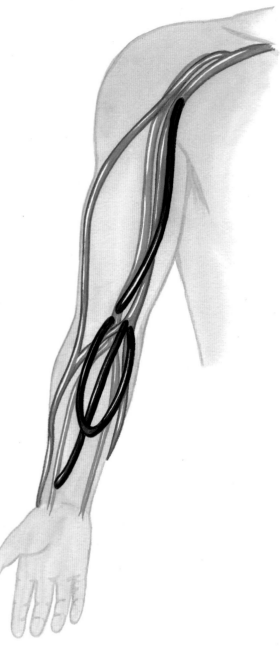

Figure 10-8. Upper extremity tunnels for arteriovenous hemoaccess.

ficial femoral artery. The dissecting finger is advanced, with a fingernail kept in contact with the arterial wall. If required, a rigid tunneling device can be used to broaden the tunnel (Fig. 10-7). Maintenance of the position behind sartorius below the quite strong musculofascial roof of the canal and anterolateral to the artery avoids any potential injury to nerve or venous structures within the canal. Damage to the saphenous nerve within the canal is a source of some morbidity to patients, and careful attention to the tunneling avoids that problem.

If required, the tunnel can be created subfascially by beginning underneath the fascia lata and extending across the sartorius into the groove between sartorius and gracilis and entering the popliteal space between sartorius and gracilis. This offers the best and lowest-risk route for the tunnel in the subfascial space. Although some surgeons prefer to use the subcutaneous space, particularly the site of harvest of the long saphenous vein, to place the tunnel, this is our least preferred option, as it is frequently a site of fluid accumulation and presents, by its nature, dead space that cannot be approximated by suture restoration. Tunnels more distal in the leg are usually the result of open dissection, and the tunnel between the popliteal space and the anterior tibial compartment has been well described in **Chapter 9**.

At the completion of all mobilizations, it has become our practice to critically review the wound and all of its components including the routes to the arteries and any tunnels formed during the exposure. We do this before performing any index operation and before any anticoagulant has been given. At the time of this review, any injuries or lymph nodes that have previously been unrecognized, or any areas of bleeding, are attended to with excision of the node and diathermy of small bleeding points and ligature of any obvious vascular or lymphatic channels. We also practice the principle that at the completion of the vascular exposure, if the index procedure in that anatomic area is not to proceed immediately, the retraction and retention should be released to prevent unnecessary pressure on the wounds when complete retraction and retention are not required for access. This is also true at the openings of tunnels, and particular care is taken with the tissues that form the orifices of the tunnel.

UPPER EXTREMITY TUNNELS FOR GRAFT ARTERIOVENOUS FISTULAS

When a direct arteriovenous fistula, such as a Cimino–Brescia fistula, is not feasible, a graft becomes necessary. Although these fistulas were initially constructed with saphenous vein as the conduit, more commonly now, synthetic materials such as PTFE are used. The aim is to provide a long access to the graft to obtain arterial blood to pass through the dialyzer and to return the venous blood to the circulation. Two common variants of these fistulas are used: radial artery to antecubital vein with the graft pursuing a straight course from distal to proximal and loop arteriovenous fistulas from the brachial artery in the elbow returning to the antecubital vein (Fig. 10-8).

The tunnel begun over the radial artery can be created with a long clamp, and, in contrast to most other subcutaneously placed grafts, it is a requirement here to have the graft superficially placed underneath the skin in the subcutaneous tissue. The other points, however, of minimum size compatible with anatomic placement of the graft and the obliteration of dead space by placement of the graft ensure firm healing and incorporation. This is essential for when the graft is used, any potential space would rapidly become filled with blood, causing perigraft hematoma.

For the loop forearm fistulas, the tunnels are created from the region of the elbow in a gentle curve down into the forearm, and a relieving counterincision is made low on the volar aspect to create the two tunnels. There is a requirement in making this tunnel to create a small flap at the region of the counterincision to allow the graft to assume its gentle curve. Subcutaneous tunnels can also be created in the upper arm and in unusual sites in emergency requirement for dialysis access; however, they do not function as effectively or with the same ease of cannulation as those present in the forearm.

Subject Index

NOTE: An *f* following a page number indicates a figure.